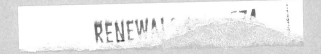

The Jossey-Bass Health Series brings together the most current information and ideas in health care from the leaders in the field. Titles from the Jossey-Bass Health Series include these essential health care resources:

Beyond Managed Care: How Consumers and Technology Are Changing the Future of Health Care, Dean C.Coddington, Elizabeth A. Fischer, Keith D. Moore, Richard L. Clarke

Board Work: Governing Health Care Organizations, Dennis D. Pointer, James E. Orlikoff

Changing the U.S. Health Care System: Key Issues in Health Services Policy and Management, Second Edition, Ronald M. Andersen, Thomas H. Rice, Gerald F. Kominski, Editors

Curing Health Care: New Strategies for Quality Improvement, Donald M. Berwick, A. Blanton Godfrey, Jane Roessner

E-Health, Telehealth, and Telemedicine: A Guide to Start-Up and Success, Marlene Maheu, Pamela Whitten, Ace Allen

Health Care 2010: The Forecast, The Challenge, Institute for the Future

Health Care in the New Millennium: Vision, Values, and Leadership, Ian Morrison

Oxymorons: The Myth of a U.S. Health Care System, J.D. Kleinke

Privacy and Confidentiality of Health Information, Jill Callahan Dennis

Strategies for the New Health Care Marketplace: Managing the Convergence of Consumerism and Technology, Dean C. Coddington, Elizabeth A. Fischer, Keith D. Moore

Technology and the Future of Health Care: Preparing for the Next 30 Years, David Ellis

The Twenty-First Century Health Care Leader, Roderick W. Gilkey, Editor, and The Center for Healthcare Leadership, Emory University School of Medicine

The CEO's Guide to Health Care Information Systems, Second Edition, Joseph M. DeLuca, Rebecca Enmark

THE STRATEGIC APPLICATION OF INFORMATION TECHNOLOGY IN HEALTH CARE ORGANIZATIONS

THE STRATEGIC APPLICATION OF INFORMATION TECHNOLOGY IN HEALTH CARE ORGANIZATIONS

SECOND EDITION

John P. Glaser

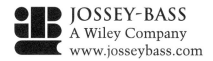

JOSSEY-BASS
A Wiley Company
www.josseybass.com

Published by

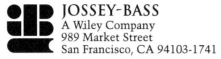

JOSSEY-BASS
A Wiley Company
989 Market Street
San Francisco, CA 94103-1741

www.josseybass.com

Jossey-Bass books and products are available through most bookstores. To contact Jossey-Bass directly, call (888) 378-2537, fax to (800) 605-2665, or visit our website at www.josseybass.com.

Substantial discounts on bulk quantities of Jossey-Bass books are available to corporations, professional associations, and other organizations. For details and discount information, contact the special sales department at Jossey-Bass.

We at Jossey-Bass strive to use the most environmentally sensitive paper stocks available to us. Our publications are printed on acid-free recycled stock whenever possible, and our paper always meets or exceeds minimum GPO and EPA requirements.

Library of Congress Cataloging-in-Publication Data

Glaser, John (John P.)
    The strategic application of information technology in health care organizations / John P. Glaser.—2nd ed.
        p. cm.—(The Jossey-Bass health series)
    Includes bibliographical references and index.
    ISBN 0-7879-5987-1 (hc : alk. paper)
    1. Health services administration—Information technology—Planning. 2. Strategic planning. I. Title. II. Series.

RA971.6.G56 2002
362.1'068'4—dc21

2001038581

SECOND EDITION
HB Printing   10 9 8 7 6 5 4 3 2 1

CONTENTS

TABLES, FIGURES, AND EXHIBITS

Tables

Figures

Exhibits

ACKNOWLEDGMENTS

The author gratefully acknowledges the contribution of Leslie Hsu to the first edition of this book, *The Strategic Application of Information Technology in Health-care Organizations* (McGraw-Hill, 1999).

ABOUT THE AUTHOR

John P. Glaser is vice president and chief information officer of Partners Health-Care System, Inc. Previously, he was vice president of Information Systems at Brigham and Women's Hospital and before that manager of the Healthcare Information Systems consulting practice at Arthur D. Little.

Glaser was the founding chairman of College of Healthcare Information Management Executives (CHIME) and is a past president of the Healthcare Information and Management Systems Society (HIMSS).

He is a fellow of HIMSS, CHIME, and the American College of Medical Informatics. He has been awarded the John Gall Award for health care CIO of the year. Partners HealthCare has received several industry awards for its effective and innovative use of information technology.

Glaser has participated in National Academy of Sciences studies on the role of the Internet in health care and health care confidentiality and security. He is on the editorial boards of *CIO Magazine, Healthcare Informatics*, the *Journal of Biomedical Informatics*, the *Journal of Healthcare Information Management*, and *Topics in Health Information Management*. He has published more than sixty articles and a book on the strategic application of information technology in health care.

He holds a Ph.D. degree in health care information systems from the University of Minnesota.

To All Who Deliver Patient Care

INTRODUCTION

Information technology (IT) can be a critical contributor to the strategic plans of health care providers to reduce costs, respond to managed care, develop a continuum of care, manage the cost and quality of that care, and improve the quality of service to patients, payers, and physicians. However, on several fronts, the leaders of health care organizations struggle with their organizations' use of and commitment to IT.

The aggregate capital projections for these systems often convey staggering numbers: tens or at times hundreds of millions of dollars. The percentage of an organization's overall capital and operating budgets devoted to information systems appears to be increasing and is on its way to being double current percentages. Although organizational leaders understand from colleagues, consultants, and the trade press that such figures are becoming commonplace, information system capital and operating budget requests cause sticker shock, and IT allocations are often growing much faster than any other segment of the budget. Moreover, the demands for IT capital compete with other pressing capital demands: opportunities to expand the delivery system through acquisition, improve service quality through facilities improvements, or enhance the ability to deliver efficacious care through new medical technology.

Health care executives have a belief, often tenuous, that information systems will provide some form of competitive advantage and will be a major contributor to organizational strategies and plans. However, it is difficult for most executives to point to a large number of prior information system investments that have led to significant and unarguable returns to the financial and competitive performance of the organization. Even successful information investments may be difficult to defend empirically and convincingly. It may not be hard to point to examples of information system failures or significant overruns.

A study by the Millennium Health Imperative, reported by Bell (1999, p. 24) in *Modern Healthcare*, notes that

- Only 49 percent of health care CIOs feel that IT has improved the quality of care, and only 26 percent of COOs believe that this is the case
- Only 45 percent of health care executives feel that a positive return on investment on IT is "very likely"

This book is intended to improve the ability of the leaders of health care organizations to invest strategically and thoughtfully in information technology and achieve desired organizational returns. This book will not focus on the "how to" aspects of several areas of IT management (such as application system selection, project management, or development of IT service levels). This should not lead you to conclude that such topics are unimportant.

Rather the book is premised on my experiences and observations, from more than a decade as a CIO in a provider organization and as a leader in health care IT industry organizations, that a consistent and deep-rooted problem facing the industry is insufficient health care IT strategy. Cash, McFarlan, and McKenney (1992) note that there are two major categories of risk that IT investments may face (where risk is defined as failure to achieve intended objectives): conceptualization failures and implementation failures.

Conceptualization failures are failures to link the organization strategies and IT strategies adequately and to define and focus the IT initiative clearly. An example of a conceptualization failure would be an intellectually anemic response to the question "What real, measurable, and significant problems will the computerized medical record solve for us?" Conceptualization failures are almost always strategy failures.

Implementation failures occur when projects run significantly over budget or deliver a shadow of the expected capabilities or just don't work. Implementation failures are often due to strategy failures because the organization has not thought strategically about the form and characteristics of the staff, technologies, and applications that should be brought to bear on an initiative.

This book takes the perspective of the role of IT in a large provider organization, particularly the integrated delivery system. This should not preclude its usefulness for executives in other sectors of the health care industry. Those of you who are health care IT executives, industry vendors and consultants, and health care leaders with an interest and modest knowledge of IT management issues should find the book informative and stimulating.

Chapter One provides an overview of strategy. Strategy is defined, and the three major areas of health care IT that require strategy are described: linkage of IT to organizational strategies, internal organizational factors that contribute to the effectiveness of IT use, and concepts that frame the organization's view of major initiatives and new technologies. Characteristics of strategic thinking are examined.

Chapter Two discusses the linkage of IT to organizational strategy. Discussion of the use of IT to further an organization's competitive position draws on lessons learned from other industries. Strategic information systems planning is reviewed. Sample planning frameworks are presented, and lessons learned about the nature of IT planning are described.

Chapter Three examines factors, internal to the organization, that have a large influence on how well the organization applies IT. One class of factors is the IT asset, which consists of applications, technical architecture, data, IT staff, and IT governance. The importance and nature of strategies directed to advancing the asset are explored. The second class of factors is IT-centric organizational attributes, which express the relationship between the IT group and the rest of the organization. Studies that have examined this class of factors are presented, and factors shown to impede the achievement of value from IT investments are reviewed. The discussion then moves on to the limitations of industry surveys, fads, and IT evaluation methodologies.

Chapter Four focuses on examples of IT strategy. Three such examples are discussed: clinical information systems, integration, and the Internet. Drawn from the experiences of Partners HealthCare System, a large integrated delivery system, these examples illustrate the role of developing "strategic views" and bring together concepts and lessons discussed in the earlier chapters of the book.

Chapter Five presents some conclusions.

You will find that this book develops a well-integrated blend of management concepts and theories with the practical realities of implementing complex information systems in complex health care organizations. I hope you find it useful.

THE STRATEGIC APPLICATION OF INFORMATION TECHNOLOGY IN HEALTH CARE ORGANIZATIONS

CHAPTER ONE

AN OVERVIEW OF STRATEGY

Strategy, as an art, science, and practice, has been a centerpiece of management and information technology (IT) literature and discussion for many years and will remain a major management concern for the foreseeable future. Effective strategies are key determinants of organizational performance. Developing effective strategies is difficult. A plethora of approaches to assist in strategy formation have been developed over the years (Harvard Business School, 1998; Stern and Stalk, 1998).

In this chapter, we discuss the nature of strategy and the different ways in which we should apply strategy to IT in health care. The chapter will present

- A definition of strategy
- A review of competitive strategy
- A discussion of the need for IT strategy and the types of IT strategy
- Characteristics of strategic thinking

Definition of Strategy

The strategy of an organization has two major components (Henderson and Venkatraman, 1993): formulation and implementation.

Formulation

Formulation involves making decisions about the mission and goals of the organization and the activities and initiatives that it will undertake to achieve them. Formulation could involve, for example, determining the following:

- Our mission is to provide high-quality medical care.
- We have a goal of reducing the cost of care while at least preserving the quality of that care.
- One of our greatest leverage points lies in reducing inappropriate and unnecessary care.
- To achieve this goal, we will place emphasis on, for example, reducing the number of inappropriate radiology procedures.
- We will carry out initiatives that enable us to intervene at the time of procedure ordering if we need to suggest a more cost-effective modality.

We can imagine other goals directed to achieving this mission. For each goal, we can envision multiple leverage points, and for each leverage point, we may see multiple initiatives. An inverted tree that cascades from our mission to a series of initiatives would emerge.

Formulation involves understanding competing ideas and choosing between them. In our example, we could have arrived at a different set of goals and initiatives. We could have decided to improve quality with less emphasis on care costs. We could have decided to focus on reducing the cost per procedure. We could have decided to produce retrospective reports, by provider, of radiology utilization and used this feedback to lead to ordering behavior change rather than intervening at the time of ordering.

In IT, we also have a need for formulation. In keeping with an IT mission to use the technology to support improvement of the quality of care, we may have a goal to integrate our clinical application systems. To achieve this goal, we may decide to do any of the following:

- Provide a common way to access all systems (single sign-on)
- Interface existing heterogeneous systems
- Require that all applications use a common database
- Implement a common suite of clinical applications from one vendor

Implementation

Implementation involves making decisions about how we structure ourselves, acquire skills, establish organizational capabilities, and alter organizational processes in order to achieve the goals and carry out the activities that we have defined during the formulation of our strategy. For example, if we have decided to reduce care costs by reducing inappropriate procedure use, we may need to implement one or more of the following solutions:

- An organizational unit of providers with health services research training to analyze care practices and identify deficiencies
- A steering committee of clinical leadership to guide these efforts and provide political support
- A provider order entry system to provide real-time feedback on order appropriateness
- Data warehouse technologies to support the analyses of utilization

Using our clinical applications integration example, we may come to one of the following determinations:

- That we need to acquire interface engine technology, adopt HL7 standards, and form an information systems department that manages the technology and interfaces applications
- That we need to engage external consulting assistance for selection of a clinical application suite and hire a group to implement the suite

The implementation component of strategy development is not the development of project plans and budgets. Rather, it is the identification of the capabilities, capacities, and competencies that the organization will need if it is to carry out the results of the formulation component of strategy.

Observations on Strategy Definition

In IT, we "conduct strategy," whether we realize it or not, when we formulate our definition of a goal and how we will approach that goal and when we define the staff, technologies, and decision-making structures needed to implement that goal. If we do not realize that we are engaged in a set of strategic decisions, we may carry out one component—for example, formulation—but not the other—for example, implementation.

At times it may not be clear whether a particular IT strategy discussion is focused on the formulation or implementation component of strategy. At a practical level, it may be irrelevant whether a specific insightful observation is one strategic component or the other. What does matter is that both components are included and are well integrated.

One's perspective may influence whether one views a conversation as strategic or tactical. The board, having given its blessing to an overall organizational strategy, may regard an IT conversation on the related clinical information systems as a tactical conversation. From the perspective of the CIO, that same conversation may be quite strategic. The CIO may regard the conversation that the clinical information systems project team has about the approach to implementation as tactical, while the project team, rightfully so from its own perspective, views that conversation as strategic. Pragmatically, it may not be particularly worth the exercise to develop an irrefutable, perspective-invariant litmus test of whether a particular conversation is strategic or not. For this book, we adopt the perspective of the CIO and the other members of the senior IT leadership of the organization.

We can have IT strategy failures in both formulation and implementation. Formulation failures are the most serious, since they can mean that the implementation strategies, no matter how well conceived and executed, are heading down the wrong path.

Let us look at some examples of potential formulation strategy failures.

• We may decide to integrate the applications across our integrated delivery system (IDS). But our IDS isn't all that integrated. Rather, it is a loose confederation of relatively independent entities. If our strategy is to put the same system in all entities and thereby achieve integration, we may fail to match the IT view of tight integration with the IDS practice of loose integration. We may spend a lot of money and not have advanced the cause of integration.

• We may decide to implement a computer-based referral system that steers the referring physician to one of our specialists and guides the collection of patient history. This system would invoke medical management rules to determine if the referral was necessary and ensure that all of the tests that need to be done prior to the consultation have been performed. We may not realize that from the referring physician's perspective, the primary problem with the referral process is the failure of the specialist to follow up rapidly on evaluation results. Hence from the referring physician's perspective, we have solved the wrong problem.

• We may decide to construct an organizational home page to attract the consumer to our organization to receive specialty care. We may fail to recognize that in our market, decisions on where to receive care are made through discussions with primary care providers or one's neighbors. Consumers will not choose a neurosurgeon from a Web site any more readily than they would from the Yellow Pages.

In these examples, the goals may have been sound (integrate applications, improve referrals, and channel patients to our specialists), but mistakes were made in selecting the activities needed to achieve those goals.

Now let us look at some examples of potential implementation strategy failures.

- We may decide to improve the "return" from information systems investments but fail to supply analysts who can work with users to develop more rigorous analyses of possible return and also fail to follow up after implementation to see if the desired return occurred.
- We may decide to implement mission-critical clinical applications but hinder the utility of those applications because we fail to take the steps necessary to ensure a very high availability infrastructure—for example, high degrees of network redundancy and superior network management tools.
- We may decide to create an IDS-wide steering committee but not realize that the vast majority of strategy development and capital decision-making power lies in the member hospitals, and hence our committee is impotent.

In each of these cases, the activities were sound (improve the analyses of the possible return from IT investments, implement mission-critical clinical applications, and provide enterprisewide guidance on IT direction), but mistakes were made in identifying and establishing the necessary organizational skills, processes, structures, or IT capabilities.

Competitive Strategy

An important aspect of competitive strategy is identifying goals and ways to achieve those goals that are materially superior to the way that a competitor has defined them (formulation) and to develop organizational capabilities that are materially superior to the capabilities of a competitor (implementation) (Lipton, 1996). For example, our competitors and we may both decide that we need to create a network of primary care providers. However, we might believe that we can move faster and use less capital than our competition if we contract with existing providers rather than buy their practices. We and our competition may both have a mission to delivery high-quality care, but our competitor has decided to focus on selected carve-outs or "focused factories" (Herzlinger, 1997) while we attempt to create a full-spectrum care delivery capacity.

Competitive strategy should attempt to define superiority that can be sustained. For example, we may believe that if our organization moves quickly, it can capture a large network of primary care providers and limit the ability of the competition to create its own network. "First to market" can provide a sustainable advantage, although no advantage is sustainable for long periods of time.

Similarly, an integrated delivery system with access to large amounts of capital can have an advantage over a system that does not. Wealth can provide a sustainable advantage.

As an IT example of competitive formulation intended to improve care quality, while our competitor is focusing on implementing provider order entry in an effort to reduce medication errors, we are focusing on creating disease management programs.

As an IT example of competitive implementation, we may assess whether we can develop means that will enable us to implement systems faster or for less cost than our competition. For example, if we could implement systems for half the cost, because of vendor partnerships, or three times faster, because of efficient implementation decision making, than our competitors, a clear advantage, perhaps sustainable, accrues to the organization.

The Need-for-IT Strategy

There are many times in IT activities (mindful of our perspective) in which the goal, or our core approaches to achieving the goal, are not particularly strategic; strategy formulation and implementation are not needed. Replacing an inpatient pharmacy system, enhancing help desk support, and delivering word processing capabilities organizationwide, while requiring well-executed projects, do not always require that we engage in conversations of organizational goals or that we take a strategic look at organizational capabilities and skills. We would see, in these examples, discussions that involved little substantive change in our understanding of what we had to do and how we should go about doing it.

There are many times when there is little likelihood that the way we achieve the goal will create a distinct competitive advantage. For example, an organization may decide that it needs a common e-mail network for its hospitals, clinics, and physicians' offices, but it does not expect that the delivered e-mail system, or its implementation, would be so superior to a competitor's e-mail system that it confers an advantage on the organization.

Much of what IT does is not strategic, nor does it require strategic thinking. Most IT projects do not require hard looks at organizational mission, thoughtful discussions of fundamental approaches to achieving those organizational goals, or significant changes in organizational capabilities. However, the fact that not all activities are strategic should not reduce the need for the IT organization to find the best technology and continuously improve its own performance. Nonstrategic activities remain important.

Areas of IT Strategy

IT strategy is particularly important in three areas, discussed in subsequent chapters:

- Activities that establish a well-conceived linkage between organizational goals and initiatives and the IT agenda
- Initiatives designed to improve internal organizational capabilities and characteristics to enhance the ability to be effective in our application of IT—for example, creating a robust IT infrastructure or improving the relationships between IT and the rest of the organization
- Concepts that govern the approach to a class of initiatives and applications— for example, are Internet technologies viewed as enabling organizational transformation, or are they seen as a normal, incremental improvement in technology?

Developing sound strategy in these areas can be very important for one simple reason: if you define what you have to do incorrectly or partially correctly, you run the risk that significant organizational resources will be misdirected. This risk has nothing to do with how well you execute the direction you choose. Being on time, on budget, and on spec is of diminished utility if you are doing the wrong thing.

Linkage to Organizational Goals and Initiatives

Organizations develop missions, goals, and plans. At times these may not be written and have elements that are vague or volatile.

IT initiatives and capabilities, as should be the case with any organizational resource, should be directed to supporting and advancing the organization's goals and plans. IT achieves strategic alignment with the organization by ensuring that it formulates its goals, activities, and plans in a way that leverages the organization's ability to carry out its strategies. This alignment occurs through two basic mechanisms.

IT Strategies Derived from Organizational Strategies. The first mechanism involves deriving the IT agenda directly from the organization's goals and plans. For example, an organization may decide that it intends to become the low-cost provider of care. It may decide to achieve this goal through the implementation of disease management programs, the reengineering of inpatient care, and reduction of the unit costs of certain tests and procedures that it believes are inordinately expensive.

The IT strategy development centers on answering questions such as "How do we apply IT to support disease management?" The answers can range from Web-based publication of disease management protocols to data warehouse technology to assess the conformance of care practice to provider documentation systems based on protocols and provider order entry systems that guide ordering decisions based on the protocols. An organization may choose all or some of these responses and arrive at different sequences of implementation. Nonetheless, it has developed an answer to the question "What is our basic approach (formulation) to using IT to support the goal of implementing disease management?" The IT plan may define the application systems and staff that are needed to support the goals (implementation).

Most of the time, the linkage between organizational strategy and IT strategy involves organizational initiatives such as adding or changing services and products or growing market share. However, at times an organization may decide that it needs to change or add to its basic, core characteristics or culture. The organization may decide that it needs its staff to be more oriented toward care quality or service delivery or the bottom line. It may decide that it needs to decentralize decision making or to recentralize decision making. The organization may decide to improve its ability to manage knowledge, or it may not. These characteristics—and there are many others—can point to initiatives for IT.

In cases where characteristics are to be changed, IT must develop strategies that answer, for example, the question "What is our basic approach to supporting a decentralized decision-making structure?" We might answer the question by permitting decentralized choices of applications as long as those applications meet certain standards—for example, run on a common platform or support an inter-application messaging standard. We might answer the question of how we support an emphasis on knowledge management by developing an intranet service that inventories knowledge.

IT Strategies That "Create" Organizational Strategies. The second mechanism involves IT capabilities enabling the organization to consider new or to significantly alter current strategic formulations and implementations. For example, telemedicine capabilities may enable the organization to consider a strategy that it had not considered, extending the reach of its specialists around the globe, or alter its approach to achieving an existing strategy, for example, relying less on specialists visiting regional health centers and more on teleconsultation.

An extreme form of this mechanism occurs when a new technology or application suggests that very fundamental strategies of the organization, or the organization's existence, may be called into question or need to undergo significant transformation. Technologies other than IT have significantly altered the strategies of health care organizations—for example, minimally invasive surgeries and anti-biotics. Advances in genetics are likely to have a dramatic impact on organizational strategy. Although IT-induced transformation is rare in health care, it is occurring with regularity in other industries. The Internet, for example, is challenging the existence of or at least transforming a range of companies that distribute "content," such as booksellers, music stores, publishers, travel agents, and stockbrokers.

Internal Capabilities and Characteristics

Organizational effectiveness in applying IT is heavily influenced by two classes of organizational capabilities and characteristics: the IT asset and IT-centric organizational attributes.

The IT asset is composed of the various IT resources that the organization has or can obtain that are applied to further the goals, plans, and initiatives of the organization. Strategies regarding the IT asset are generally implementation strategies. The IT asset, discussed in more detail in Chapter Three, has five components:

- *Applications,* which are the systems that users interact with—for example, scheduling, billing, and computerized record systems
- *Technical architecture,* consisting of the base technology—for example, networks, operating systems, and workstations that form the foundation for applications and the approaches adopted to ensure that these technologies "fit together"
- *Data,* which refers to all the organization's data and analysis and access technologies
- *IT staff,* the analysts, programmers, and computer operators who, day in and day out, manage and advance information systems in an organization, along with the IT organization structure, core competencies, and IT organization characteristics such as agility
- *IT governance,* which consists of the organizational mechanisms by which IT priorities are set, IT policies and procedures are developed, and IT management responsibility is distributed

When a very explicit effort is made to link IT strategies to organizational strategies, activities directed toward altering the IT asset can result. The organization's strategy may call for new applications, development of more reliable infrastructure, or the creation of new departments, such as quality measurement. Often, however, the need to develop strategies for the IT asset cuts across organizational plans and activities. For example, strategies may be developed that alter the asset as a response to questions such as these:

- What is our approach to ensuring that our infrastructure is more agile?
- What is our approach to attracting and retaining superb IT talent?
- How do we improve our prioritization of IT initiatives?
- Is there a way we can significantly improve the impact of our clinical information systems on our care processes?

A variety of studies, discussed in Chapter Three, have identified IT-centric organizational attributes that appear to have a significant influence on the effectiveness of an organization in applying IT. These factors include the following:

- The relationship between the IT group and the rest of the organization
- The presence of top management support for IT
- Organizational comfort with "visionary" IT applications
- Organizational experience with IT

These factors, which are different from the IT asset, can be created or changed. If creation or change is desired, strategies will have to be developed.

Concepts That Frame the IT Challenge

There are classes of technology, applications, or management techniques that can appear to have the potential for a significant impact on our industry, organizations, and the way we implement and apply information systems. Examples today include the Internet, component-based architectures, knowledge management, and computerized medical record systems.

It may not be initially clear how these "technologies" will further organizational strategies or the impact, if adopted, on the IT asset. As organizations adopt or explore these kinds of technologies, they develop formulation and implementation concepts that guide how they think about the technology, which in turn has great influence over whether and how they will adopt it, how they approach the implementation, and how they will evaluate the technology's success. For example, there are several ways to think about the Internet and its technologies:

- As a "universal" presentation layer allowing access to a diverse array of legacy systems by a diverse array of workstations
- As a means to publish organizational knowledge
- As a means to find services and information offered by others

- As a means to extend an organization's services into the home
- As a replacement for electronic data interchange (EDI)
- As an approach to the alteration of a distribution channel—for example, ordering your PC directly from the manufacturer rather than from the local distributor

All of these views are "correct" in that all can be effective. However, once an organization chooses a concept, it tends to think about the technology in that way, often to the exclusion of other approaches. Moreover, the organization's concept can be wrong or ineffectual. For example, if an organization viewed Internet technologies solely as the universal front end, it would miss an extraordinary set of other opportunities for the technology.

Concepts that frame the IT challenge will be discussed in more detail in Chapter Four.

Characteristics of Strategic Thinking

Strategic thinking and discussion have several characteristics.

- Strategic thinking centers on discussions of core concepts and ideas that lead to the determination of goals and initiatives (formulation) and the definition of organizational capabilities and competencies needed (implementation) if we are to implement those goals and initiatives.
- The consequences of being wrong are generally serious. An application software company that had a strategy that did not include the Internet revolution is generally paying dearly for that strategy. Several health care provider organizations have been badly damaged by failed integrated delivery network strategies.
- A strategic decision has clear and illuminating ramifications for many other decisions. For example, an organization can decide that a critical component of a clinical information system is the introduction of decision support that guides a provider's decisions on ordering and referring. Such a strategy tells the organization that a provider order entry application and medical logic processors are critical aspects of its clinical system infrastructure. The organization would know that it needs a group of physicians and organizational processes to develop and monitor decision rules. The organization would know that it needs to code data for medications, lab tests, procedures, and problems since these form the basis for many rules. These decisions and calls fall naturally from a strategy of centering on decision support.

• Strategic decisions often imply relatively significant changes in how business is conducted. Strategic decisions often involve changes in the core concepts that guide organizational activity. Any time the concepts that underlie an organization undergo fundamental change, the organization's activities, market position, processes, and structure can undergo significant change. For example, a move to protocol-driven care, adoption of risk arrangements, and the creation of a continuum of care all involve the adoption of new organizational concepts and will necessitate some level of fundamental change. Similarly, the IT organization can experience significant change as a result of strategic decisions such as moving to Internet-based architectures or investing heavily in computerized medical records.

• The implementation of strategic decisions will require significant resources and intense political activity. Extensive resource commitments and political activity are the natural consequence and antecedent of the introduction of major organizational change.

• Strategies take time, multiple iterations, and lots of analysis to develop, and they must be monitored. Organizations rarely fully understand either the consequences of their strategies or the complete set of organizational activities and investments required to implement them. Strategies can be wrong or "off by 15 degrees." The organization learns as it adjusts itself and assesses the effectiveness of its strategies.

• In IT, we often confuse tactical decisions with strategic decisions. "Should we use applications that are browser-based?" is not a strategic question. The question needs a formulation or implementation strategic context before it can be answered. One might be able to arrive at the browser question through a line of reasoning as follows:

1. A major goal in our development of our technical architecture is the creation of the attribute of architectural agility (formulation).
2. We would define agility (a framing concept) as the ability to change a major component of our architecture without having to change other components of our architecture (formulation).
3. If we could run complex applications in a way that essentially ignores (or need not be aware of) the client operating system, we would have established some reasonably high level of agility, since we could change clients and client operating systems without having to change the applications (formulation).
4. To the degree that browser-based applications provide such agility, we should pursue them (implementation).
5. If we pursue this technology, we will need, among other things, Web development expertise and a secure Web infrastructure (implementation).

Unless one has started from some level of strategic thinking, it is hard to give a good answer to the browser-based application question.

Nor can one directly answer the question "Should we computerize the patient record?" One has to ask and answer the question "What is our basic approach to applying the technology to improve care?" If the answer is "We must improve the accessibility of patient data and improve the comprehensiveness of patient documentation," one is in a position to assess whether the computerized patient record is a solid approach to improving care.

Summary

It is crucial that health care organizations apply strategic thinking, questioning, and analysis to their investments in information technology. Strategic thinking requires that we pursue fundamental questions regarding the formulation of goals and the activities needed to achieve those goals. Strategic thinking requires that we pursue fundamental implementation questions such as the need to add or change core organizational capabilities.

Strategic thinking should be applied during conversations that link IT investments to organizational initiatives, development of plans to improve internal IT capabilities, and the framing of our view of major classes of technology, applications, or management techniques.

Strategic thinking has several characteristics, and organizations can confuse a strategic question with a tactical question.

Not all conversations are strategic conversations. Not all IT investments are strategic investments. Classifying a tactical conversation, regardless of its importance, as strategic does not enhance the quality of the conversation.

CHAPTER TWO

LINKAGE OF IT STRATEGY TO ORGANIZATIONAL STRATEGY

Information technology can support and at times be a critical contributor to effecting organizational strategies. Efforts to improve care quality can require clinical information systems and databases to analyze patterns of care. The integration of the integrated delivery system (IDS) can be advanced through the development of a common e-mail platform, a clinical data repository, and an enterprise master person index.

Information technology can enable the organization to consider new elements and aspects of its strategy. The organization could use the Internet as a way of reaching consumers with health information and providing access to the organization's health services. Provider order entry systems can be used to proactively guide medication decisions as a way of effecting protocol-driven care and reducing medication errors.

In this chapter, we explore this linkage between organizational strategies and IT strategies. We will cover two major topics:

- IT strategic planning frameworks and methodologies
- Lessons learned from efforts to apply IT as a "competitive weapon"

Strategic IT Planning Frameworks and Methodologies

The IT strategic planning process has several objectives:

- To ensure that information technology plans and activities align with the plans and activities of the organization; in other words, the IT needs of each aspect of organizational strategy are clear, and the portfolio of IT plans and activities can be mapped to organizational strategies and operational needs

- To ensure that the alignment is comprehensive; in other words,

    Each aspect of strategy has been addressed from an IT perspective recognizing that not all aspects have an IT component and not all components will be funded.

    The non-IT organizational initiatives needed to ensure maximum leverage of the IT initiative (for example, process reengineering) are understood.

    The organization has not missed a strategic IT opportunity, such as those that might result from new technologies.
- To develop a tactical plan that details approved project descriptions, timetables, budgets, staffing plans, and plan risk factors
- To create a communication tool that can inform the organization of the IT initiatives that will be undertaken and those that will not
- To establish a political process that helps ensure that the plan results have sufficient organizational support

Despite the simplicity implied by these statements, the development of well-aligned IT strategies has been notoriously difficult for many years, and there appears to be no reason that such an alignment will become significantly easier over time.

Over the course of the years, several methodologies have been developed in an effort to assist the organization in its effort to develop well-aligned IT plans. There are two major types of methodologies:

- Those that use assessments of a specific organization's environment, strategies, missions, and goals and from that derive the related IT plans
- Those that arrive at IT plans based on very fundamental views of the nature of organizations and their processes and the nature of forces such as competition

In both types, the methodologies assist in developing organizational support, serve to communicate the plan, and lead to the eventual tactical plans of projects, timetables, and budgets.

Derived IT Linkage

Most IT planning methodologies used in health care today derive the IT plan from a thorough review of the organization's external environment, mission, goals, strategies, capabilities, and immediate competitive position. Three such methodologies are presented here.

Generic Methodology. A generic IT strategic planning methodology is depicted in Figure 2.1.

In this methodology, interviews are conducted, often by consultants, to review organizational plans and strategies with organizational leadership and

FIGURE 2.1. GENERIC IT STRATEGIC PLANNING METHODOLOGY.

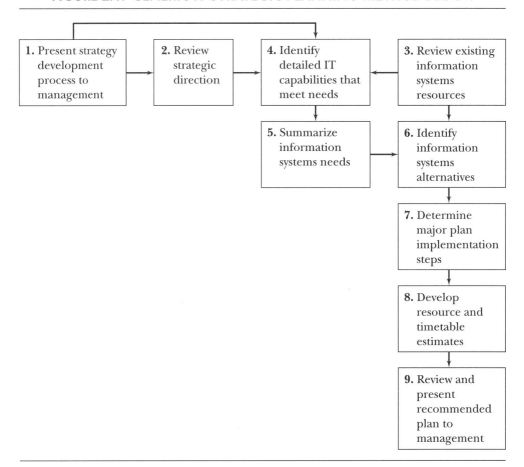

define operational needs with middle management. A portfolio of application and technical infrastructure needs is developed. Current IT resources are surveyed, and the gap between those resources and the needed resources is determined. Priorities are defined, and budgets, timetables, and projects are eventually developed. These methodologies also include provisions and support for the formation of committees, to ensure broad input and garner political support for the plan's conclusions, and the delivery of sets of data that can limit the need of the organization to engage in original data gathering (for example, the average costs of implementing a particular type of application system).

Minard Methodology. The annual planning cycle presented by Minard (1991) offers a strategy of reevaluation, modification, and evolution of ideas or issues. The cycle is presented in Figure 2.2.

FIGURE 2.2. MINARD MODEL.

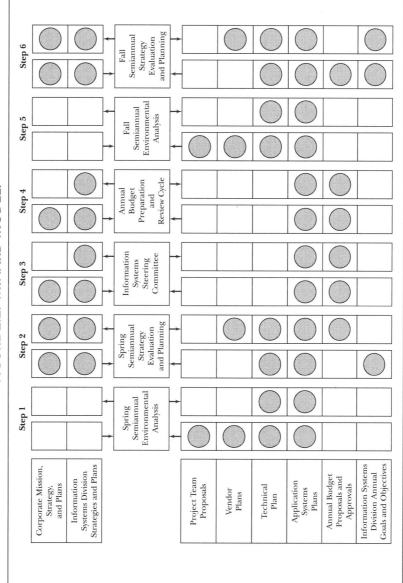

Source: Used with permission from *Health Care Computer Systems for the 1990s: Critical Executive Decisions* by Bernie Minard (Chicago: Health Administration Press, 1991), p. 46.

There are six steps to the annual planning cycle. Arrows pointing into the rectangle represent plans and issues that are reviewed and analyzed, and arrows pointing out of the rectangle represent plans that are being updated. The shaded circles indicate planning items that correspond to the step.

The first step in the annual planning cycle is the "Spring Semiannual Environmental Analysis," which involves reevaluation of new IT opportunities. The analysis can take place through conferences or presentations by vendors, consultants, hospital managers, and technical experts. Data analysis, data gathering, and learning experiences occur at this level, and proposed alterations to application system plans are recorded.

The second step is the "Spring Semiannual Strategy Evaluation and Planning," which requires participants to review proposed changes in corporate, information system, technical, and application system plans. Consensus is vital at this stage.

Step 3 involves the meeting of the "Information Systems Steering Committee," the highest-level executive group. The committee meets to review and approve proposed IT plans.

Step 4 is the "Annual Budget Preparation and Review Cycle," where budget items are approved and planned projects become planned objectives for the following year.

Step 5 is the "Fall Semiannual Environmental Analysis," which repeats the procedures of step 1.

Step 6 is the "Fall Semiannual Strategy Evaluation and Planning," which repeats procedures of step 2. Goals and objectives for the coming year are finalized and divided among project teams or individuals.

Component Alignment Model. The Component Alignment Model (CAM) (Martin, Wilkins, and Stawski, 1998) is based on the premise that strategic IT planning requires that the organization adopt a systems mentality where it sees itself as part of a larger environment and context rather than as a confederation of individual business units. CAM consists of seven components, which are grouped into two major sets: controllable components and controllable components. CAM is presented in Figure 2.3.

Uncontrollable components (external environment and emerging information technologies) cannot be affected by an organization's strategic plans, while controllable components (organization infrastructure and processes, mission, IT infrastructure and processes, business strategy, and IT strategy) can be directly affected by an organization's strategic plan.

The external environment component describes everything that occurs outside of the organization's corporate environment—for example, mergers and affiliations, public perception of the health care environment, and federal regulation and reimbursement. The emerging information technology component describes

FIGURE 2.3. COMPONENT ALIGNMENT MODEL.

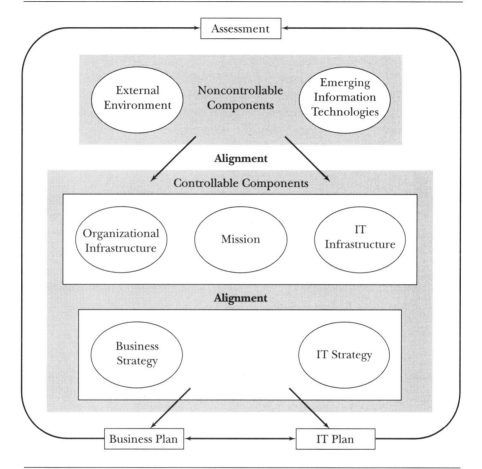

Source: Adapted with permission from J. Martin, A. Wilkins, and S. Stawski, "The Component Alignment Model: A New Approach to Health Care Information Technology Strategic Planning," in vol. 19, no. 1 of *Topics in Health Information Management,* p. 8, © 1998 Aspen Publishers, Inc.

any new technologies currently being developed, such as applications based on Web architectures. The organizational infrastructure and processes component describes an organization's services and management structures and philosophies—for example, whether the organization emphasizes patient-focused or department-focused care. The mission component describes the main goals or objectives of the organization. The IT infrastructure and processes component describes the software, hardware, and personnel being used currently as a resource for delivering IT services. Business strategy describes an organization's business strategy—for example, downsizing or developing centers of excellence in specialty areas. IT strategy describes an organization's IT goals, objectives, and strategic plans.

All of the components are interdependent and must be coordinated in response to changes in the health care industry and organizational direction. Each component needs to undergo continuous reassessment and modification known as alignment. There are two types of alignment: unidirectional and multidimensional. Unidirectional alignment is the alignment of controllable components in response to changes in the uncontrollable components. Multidimensional alignment occurs between the five controllable components.

The CAM process defines each component and seeks to establish alignment through three phases: assessment, visioning, and plan development.

Linkage Based on Fundamental Views

Several IT strategic planning methodologies are based on fundamental views of the nature of organizations and organizational processes and the nature of competition. Often these views are originally presented in literature that examines management and strategy issues in general and then are adapted for use in IT strategic planning. For example, Porter's work on competitive forces (1980) was subsequently adapted by McFarlan (1984) for use in IT planning. Three examples of IT linkage based on fundamental views are discussed here.

The Value Chain. A useful framework for analyzing the strategic significance of information technology is the "value chain" described by Porter and Millar (1985). The value chain is a system of interdependent activities connected by linkages. The value chain divides company activities, called "value activities," into the technologically and economically distinct activities it performs to do business. The value chain is depicted in Figure 2.4.

Value activities must be performed at a lower cost, or lead to differentiation and a premium price, in order for a company to gain competitive advantage. These activities fall into nine categories that are summarized into two overall activities. Primary activities are those that are involved in the physical creation of the product, such as inbound logistics, operations, outbound logistics, marketing and sales, and service, while support activities are those that provide inputs and infrastructure and allow primary activities to take place, such as firm infrastructure, human resource management, technology development, and procurement.

Linkages occur when the way in which one activity is performed affects the cost or effectiveness of other activities. Effective development of linkages can be a very powerful source of competitive advantage—a good example is the efficiencies gained through just-in-time deliveries of supplies.

Companies can differ in the competitive scope or breadth of their activities, with scope being a potential source of competitive advantage. Competitive scope

FIGURE 2.4. THE VALUE CHAIN.

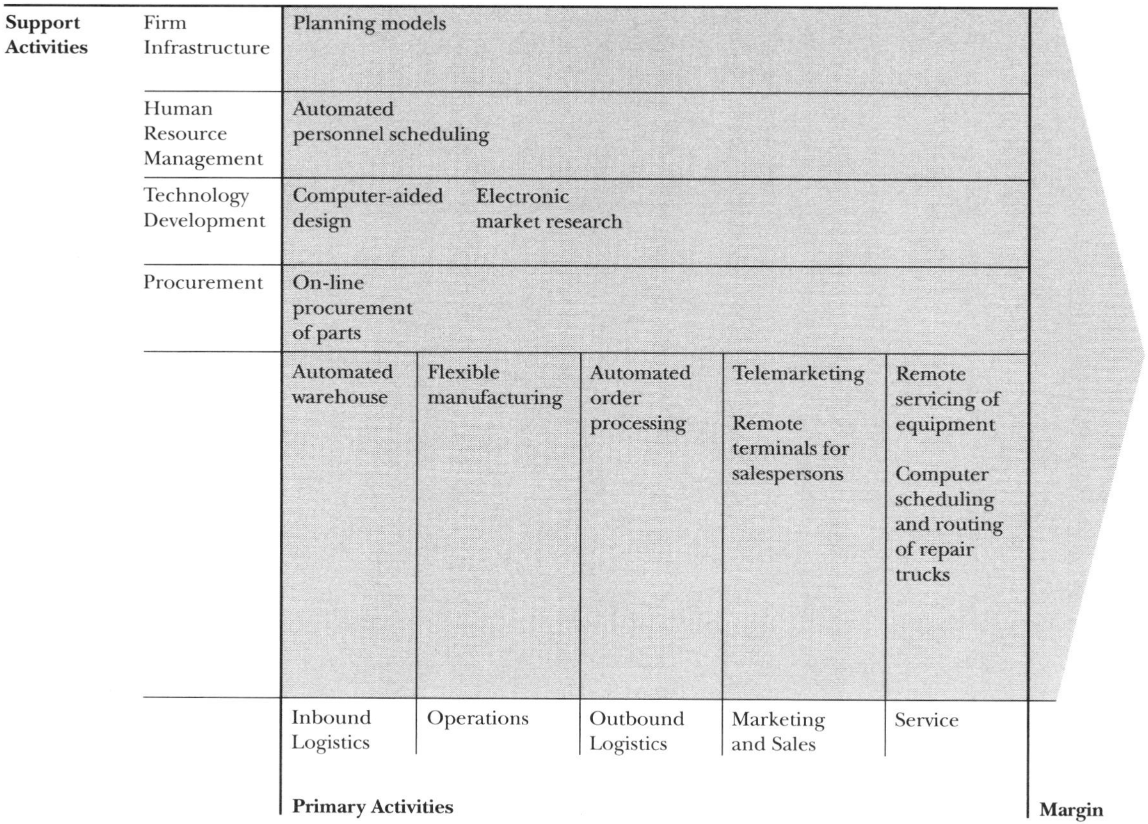

Support Activities	Firm Infrastructure	Planning models				
	Human Resource Management	Automated personnel scheduling				
	Technology Development	Computer-aided design	Electronic market research			
	Procurement	On-line procurement of parts				
		Automated warehouse	Flexible manufacturing	Automated order processing	Telemarketing Remote terminals for salespersons	Remote servicing of equipment Computer scheduling and routing of repair trucks
		Inbound Logtistics	Operations	Outbound Logistics	Marketing and Sales	Service
		Primary Activities				

Margin

Source: Reprinted by permission of *Harvard Business Review.* Exhibit 3 from "How Information Gives You a Competitive Advantage" by Michael E. Porter and Victor E. Millar, July-Aug. 1985. Copyright © 1985 by the Harvard Business School Publishing Corporation.

ranges from broad to narrow scope. An organization can potentially serve more industries or geographical areas by performing more activities internally; in other words, an organization does not need to establish relationships with others in several regions in order to perform the activities. An organization can narrow scope by tailoring the value chain to a specific product, buyer, or geographical region.

Porter and Millar (1985) note that information technology has gained strategic significance because it is constantly transforming linkages, the way value activities are performed, and the competitive scope. For every value activity, there is an information processing unit, which stores, manipulates, and transmits any data needed to perform the value activity, and a physical processing unit, which includes all physical tasks required to perform the value activity. Information technology is transforming both of these units, making information processes cost less and physical processes faster, more accurate, and more flexible. Information technology can also alter competitive scope by allowing companies to coordinate value activities in distant geographical locations. Figure 2.4 maps a series of IT applications for a manufacturing organization to their possible contribution to components of the value chain

In health care, we might define such activities broadly, for example, patient access, and narrowly, for example, dispense medication. Linkages can include procedure orders, referrals, and eligibility determination.

An organization might decide to compete on the basis of the value activity of access, for example, by enabling a patient to get an appointment within twenty-four hours of request. This strategy would quickly lead one to conclude that certain applications, such as computerized medical records and patient-provider communication applications, were critical. A strategy that focused on the value activity of second opinions would lead to a conclusion of referral and diagnostic imaging applications.

The value chain approach to IT strategic planning is very different from one that starts with a reading of the organization's strategic plan. One identifies the IT strategy by defining value activities and linkages that can be improved or altered rather than through a direct examination of the organization's strategy.

Competitive Forces. The competitive forces model (Porter, 1980) examines forces that shape the competitive environment and hence an industry's—and its member organizations'—profitability. Porter identifies five competitive forces that determine an industry's profitability: the bargaining power of buyers, the bargaining power of suppliers, the threat of new entrants, the threat of substitute products, and the rivalry among existing competitors. To gain competitive advantage, companies must devise methods to counter each of these forces. Figure 2.5 presents an updated version of the competitive forces model that illustrates the potential effects of the Internet on these forces (Porter, 2001).

FIGURE 2.5. HOW THE INTERNET INFLUENCES INDUSTRY STRUCTURE.

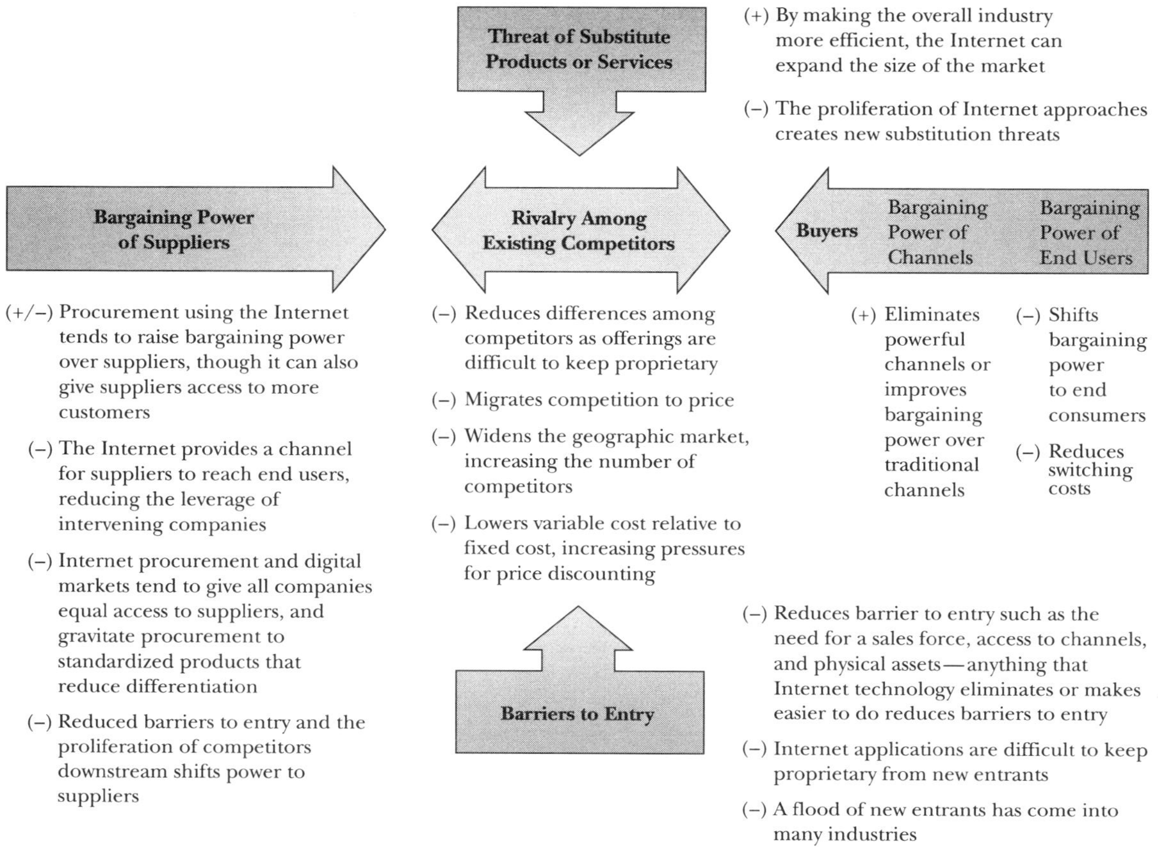

Threat of Substitute Products or Services

(+) By making the overall industry more efficient, the Internet can expand the size of the market

(−) The proliferation of Internet approaches creates new substitution threats

Bargaining Power of Suppliers

(+/−) Procurement using the Internet tends to raise bargaining power over suppliers, though it can also give suppliers access to more customers

(−) The Internet provides a channel for suppliers to reach end users, reducing the leverage of intervening companies

(−) Internet procurement and digital markets tend to give all companies equal access to suppliers, and gravitate procurement to standardized products that reduce differentiation

(−) Reduced barriers to entry and the proliferation of competitors downstream shifts power to suppliers

Rivalry Among Existing Competitors

(−) Reduces differences among competitors as offerings are difficult to keep proprietary

(−) Migrates competition to price

(−) Widens the geographic market, increasing the number of competitors

(−) Lowers variable cost relative to fixed cost, increasing pressures for price discounting

Buyers

Bargaining Power of Channels

(+) Eliminates powerful channels or improves bargaining power over traditional channels

Bargaining Power of End Users

(−) Shifts bargaining power to end consumers

(−) Reduces switching costs

Barriers to Entry

(−) Reduces barrier to entry such as the need for a sales force, access to channels, and physical assets—anything that Internet technology eliminates or makes easier to do reduces barriers to entry

(−) Internet applications are difficult to keep proprietary from new entrants

(−) A flood of new entrants has come into many industries

The model can be used to evaluate how information technology can alter each of these competitive forces (McFarlan, 1984). For example, the bargaining power of buyers may be increased by electronic catalogues and consumer-oriented quality-rating Web sites. Barriers to new entrants in some industries have increased due to the large investments that need to be spent to remain on the cutting edge of technology; for example, organizations often join integrated delivery systems because of the capital costs of the information technology that is viewed as necessary in order to compete. The Internet can reduce the role of traditional channels (such as the referring physician, a buyer of specialty services) by supporting a patient's finding and accessing a specialist. Internet-based health insurance companies, often focusing on supporting a movement to defined contributions, can be viewed by a traditional payer as a threat, a source of substitute products.

Information technology can also create competitive advantage by lowering costs, enhancing differentiation, and changing competitive scope, all of which minimize the potential for substitute products. IT can enable the creation of new industries and new businesses—Internet-based health care consumer content, health insurance products, providers of second opinions—all of which alter the rivalry force.

Porter and Millar (1985) offer IT managers five steps for taking advantage of IT:

1. Assess information intensity, in other words, how essential and pervasive information processing is generally in the industry.
2. Determine the role of information technology in industry structure; in other words, to what degree has IT led to the current industry structure? International banking is an example of an industry whose current form has been significantly shaped by IT.
3. Identify and rank the ways in which information technology might create a competitive advantage—for example, by providing referring physicians with access to a specialist's schedule.
4. Investigate how information technology might spawn new businesses, such as the examination of disease management as a business by pharmaceutical companies.
5. Develop a plan for taking advantage of information technology.

There are many places in health care where IT can alter competitive forces. IT enables providers to assume full delegation under capitation. Management of delegation would be effectively impossible without IT. Delegation alters the power between the supplier (the managed care company) and the buyer (the provider). Telemedicine can act as a means to provide a substitute product wherein one provider "invades" the market of another provider with a different approach to obtaining access to specialists. Many health care provider organizations are attempting to strengthen their relationships with their buyers (referring physicians) by providing real-time access to information about the referring physician's patient's hospital care. Consumer access to Internet-based provider report cards and quality measures strengthens their power as buyers.

As with the value change analysis, the process of arriving at an IT strategic plan using the competitive forces framework has a very different conversation than the one that centers on the published organizational strategic plan.

E-Opportunities. Feeny (2001) presents a framework that enables organizations to construct a coherent map of strategic opportunities to apply Web-based technologies. The model notes that the Internet can be the impetus to rethink existing business models, processes, and partner relationships. Unlike the other two models, the e-opportunities framework starts with an information technology perspective.

The model outlines three categories of opportunities; operations, marketing, and customer services. E-operations opportunities involve the use of Web-based technologies to effect fundamental change in the way an organization manages itself and its supply chain. E-marketing opportunities focus on activities such as direct interaction with a customer or through a distribution channel. E-service opportunities can enable an organization to enact new ways to address customer needs. Figure 2.6 provides an overview of the e-opportunities framework.

For health care organizations, e-operations opportunities may take several forms:

- Internet-based supply purchasing—for example, pooling of supply requests for proposals by several organizations in order to increase purchase volume
- Prescription writing, formulary checking, and interaction checking using handheld devices

E-marketing opportunities, too, may take several forms:

- Delivery of consumer health content and wellness management tools over the Internet
- Use of consumer health profiles to suggest disease management and wellness programs

E-service opportunities could take these forms:

- Patient-provider communication and transaction applications
- Web-based applications to support the clinical conversation between referring and consulting physicians

FIGURE 2.6. THE THREE E-OPPORTUNITY DOMAINS AND THEIR COMPONENTS.

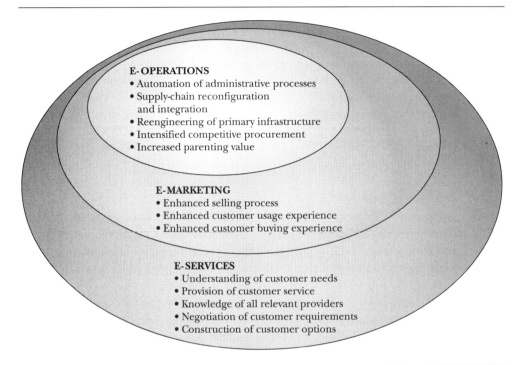

E-OPERATIONS
- Automation of administrative processes
- Supply-chain reconfiguration and integration
- Reengineering of primary infrastructure
- Intensified competitive procurement
- Increased parenting value

E-MARKETING
- Enhanced selling process
- Enhanced customer usage experience
- Enhanced customer buying experience

E-SERVICES
- Understanding of customer needs
- Provision of customer service
- Knowledge of all relevant providers
- Negotiation of customer requirements
- Construction of customer options

Source: Reprinted from "Making Business Sense of the E-Opportunity" by David Feeny, *MIT Sloan Management Review,* Winter 2001, Vol. 42, No. 2, p.42, by permission of the publisher. Copyright © 2001 by MIT Sloan Management Review Association. All rights reserved.

A specific opportunity may support more than one opportunity category. The strength of an opportunity will depend on the following factors:

- Level of information content in the product—for example, the treatment of an asthmatic has a high level of information content as part of the "treatment product"
- Information density along the supply chain—for example, the "supply chain" involved in managing a patient with congestive heart failure has a high information density
- Information dispersion—for example, a large number of providers may (or may not) be involved in the care of a patient

Observations on IT Frameworks and Planning

Processes and methodologies that help organizations develop IT plans, whether based on derived linkage or the examination of more fundamental characteristics of organizations, can be very helpful. If well executed, they can do all of the following:

- Lead to the identification of a portfolio of IT applications and initiatives that are well linked to the organization's strategy
- Identify alternatives and approaches that might not have been understood without the process
- Contribute to a more thorough analyses of the major aspects of the plan
- Enhance and ensure necessary leadership participation and support
- Help the organization be more decisive
- Ensure that the allocation of resources among competing alternative is rational and politically defensible
- Enhance communication of the developed plan

Persistence of the Alignment Problem. Despite the presence of frameworks and large numbers of academic and consultant examinations of the topic, the IT alignment issue has been a top concern of senior leadership for several decades. The annual Computer Science Corporation survey of IT management issues finds that aligning IT with the rest of the organization has been a top concern for several years in a row. There are several reasons for the persistent difficulty in achieving alignment (Bensaou and Earl, 1998):

- Business strategies are often unclear or volatile.
- IT opportunities are poorly understood.
- The different parts of the organization have different priorities.

Weill and Broadbent (1998) note that effective IT alignment requires that organizational leaders understand clearly and integrate, strategically and tactically, the following four domains:

- The organization's strategic context, in other words, its strategies and market position
- The organization's environment
- The IT strategy
- The IT portfolio, for example, the current applications, technology, and staff skills

Understanding and integrating these four complex and continuously evolving areas is exceptionally difficult.

Two more reasons could be added to these lists of factors that make alignment difficult. For one thing, the organization may find that it has not achieved the gains, apparently achieved by others, that it has heard or read about, nor have the promises of the vendors of the technologies materialized. Organizations often view these gaps between expectations and results as an alignment problem. Another difficulty is that often the value of IT, particularly infrastructure, is difficult to quantify. IT can also be expensive. Alignment can refer to the challenge of assessing the value of IT investment opportunities. Both these factors will be discussed in more detail in Chapter Three.

The Limitations of Alignment. As we shall also see in Chapter Three, although alignment is important, it will not guarantee effective organizational application of IT. Planning methodologies cannot, by themselves, overcome other factors that, if weak, can significantly diminish the likelihood that IT investments will lead to improved organizational performance. These factors include poor relationships between IT staff and the rest of the organization, inadequate technical infrastructure, and ill-conceived IT governance mechanisms.

IT planning methodologies also cannot overcome unclear strategies or necessarily compensate for material competitive weaknesses.

Superb alignment techniques will not turn an organization that is limited in its ability to apply IT effectively into one that is brilliant at IT use. In an analogous fashion, if one has mediocre painting skills, a class on painting technique will make one a better painter but will not turn one into Picasso. Perhaps this reason, more than any other, is why alignment remains persistently as a top-ranked IT issue. Organizations are searching for excellence in the wrong place; it cannot be delivered purely by methodology.

Alignment at Maturity. Organizations that have a history of IT excellence would appear to evolve to a state where their alignment process is "methodology-less." A study by Earl (1993) of organizations in the United Kingdom that had a history of IT excellence found that their IT planning processes had several significant characteristics.

• IT planning was not a separate process. IT planning, and the strategic discussion of IT, occurred as an integral part of organizational strategic planning processes and management discussions. In these organizations, management did not think of separating out an IT discussion during the course of strategy development, any more than it would run a separate finance or human resource planning processes. IT planning was an unseverable, intertwined component of the normal management conversation. This would suggest that there is no separate IT steering committee.

- IT planning had neither a beginning nor an end. Often IT planning processes start in one month every year and are done, for example, three months later. In the studied organizations, the IT planning and strategy conversation went on all of the time. This does not mean that an organization doesn't have to have a temporally demarcated process designed to form a budget every year. Rather it means that IT planning is a continuous process reflecting the continuous change in the environment and organizational plans and strategies.

- IT planning involved shared decision making and shared learning between IT and the organization. IT leadership informed organizational leadership of the potential contribution of new technologies and constraints of current technologies. Organizational leadership ensured that IT leadership understood the business plans and strategies and constraints. The IT budget and annual tactical plan resulted from a shared analysis and set of conclusions.

- The IT plan emphasized themes. Weill and Broadbent (1998) would refer to a theme as a "maxim." Examples of maxims would be "develop partnerships with customers on a worldwide basis" and "pursue cost reduction relentlessly." A provider organization may have themes of improving care quality, reducing costs, and integrating the delivery system. During the course of any given year, it will have initiatives that are intended to advance the organization along these themes. The mixture of initiatives will change from year to year, but the themes endure over the course of many years. Themes serve as basis for criteria for choosing between alternative "foundational" activities. Themes, such as care improvement, help organizations understand the need for foundation initiatives such as the establishment of a group to measure care quality or the standardization on common vocabularies for clinical data. Themes provide a basis for crafting technical architecture; for example, infrastructure reliability and performance become exceptionally important if significant multiyear investments will be made in systems to be used directly by care providers.

Summarizing Earl's work would suggest that mature IT alignment, as it occurs in the course of normal management conversation, is iterative and ongoing; focuses on core, strategic themes; has short time horizons for initiatives; and is conducted by the same senior management in the same conversations that decide and develop strategies overall.

Summary

IT strategic planning methodologies and frameworks can be very helpful. They can provide a needed discipline and process. They can help organizational leadership "see" new IT opportunities.

In practice, both types of methodologies should be used. The IT strategy should be derivable from the specifics of the overall organizational strategy. However, organizations should also step back from the perhaps "normal" mode of strategy development and assess their strategy using a framework based on a more fundamental understanding of industries and competition. Whether e-opportunities or competitive forces or value chain analysis is used is less important than the exercise of assessing strategy from the perspective of a fundamental view of an industry and its dynamics.

However, alignment remains a difficult challenge, and these methodologies and frameworks are not a panacea; they will not overcome other organizational limitations.

It appears that organizations that have reached maturity in their IT use have evolved these alignment processes to the point where they are no longer distinguishable as separate processes. This observation should not be construed as advice to cease using such methodologies or disband effective steering committees. Such an evolution, to the degree that it is normative—for example, kids will grow up (at least most of them will)—may occur naturally.

Information Technology as a Competitive Weapon

As organizations examine strategies and capabilities, an entirely reasonable question is "Can the application of information technology provide a competitive advantage to an organization?"

Over the past two decades, across a wide range of industries, answers to this question have been explored. Answers continue to come forward, developed most recently through the lens of the Internet (see Porter, 2001). Perhaps as a result of continued evolution of the technology and continued transformation of industries and economies, answers will always be sought and found.

Here we will review the experiences of several non–health care organizations in which information technology has appeared to provide a competitive advantage. These cases have withstood the scrutiny of time. We will also discuss lessons learned and answers developed to the question regarding competitive advantage.

Case Studies

Several superb examples of the use of IT to achieve a competitive advantage have been developed, documented, and studied (McKenney, Copeland, and Mason, 1995). We will take a look at three examples; the American Airlines SABRE system, the American Hospital Supply's ASAP system, and a set of systems implemented by Federal Express. Lessons from each of these cases will also be summarized.

SABRE. The American Airlines reservation system, known as SABRE, is regarded as one of the legendary examples of the competitive use of IT. The development of SABRE can be traced back to the late 1940s. American Airlines was seeking to address operational issues and inefficiencies associated with the manual keeping of records of flight manifests. By the mid-1970s, SABRE was providing travel agents with the ability to book airline flights interactively. SABRE, the name of the reservation system, eventually became the name of a business.

American Airlines is today a world leader in electronic distribution and information technology solutions for travel and travel-related services. SABRE provides its clients with travel reservation automation, advanced decision-support systems, customized software development and software products, transaction processing, systems integration, consulting, and information technology outsourcing. Clients include travel agencies, airlines, railroads, lodging companies, transportation services, oil and gas companies, and the financial services industry.

SABRE handles over 45 million fares in the database, 40 million changes each month, and 2,000 messages per second, and it creates more than 500,000 passenger name records every day (Hopper, 1990). More than 130,000 terminals in travel agencies link to SABRE. SABRE also manages 200,000 personal computers, 45,370 telephone numbers, and 10,200 voice mailboxes. In 1990, it was the world's largest privately owned real-time computer system.

American Airlines had five strategic objectives for SABRE in 1982 (McKenney, Copeland, and Mason, 1995):

- Display American's flights before those of competitors; for example, if an agent wanted to book a flight from Boston to Los Angeles, SABRE would list the American Airlines offerings first
- Maintain SABRE as the industry leader among automated airline reservations systems
- Receive revenue from every reservation made by subscribers to SABRE regardless of the carrier chosen for the flight
- Derive revenue from other carriers who use the SABRE system
- Ensure that SABRE generated a satisfactory return on investment without consideration of incremental passenger revenues

It is difficult to question the success of SABRE. By 1983, American had captured 27 percent of automated travel agent locations and accounted for 43 percent of the travel revenues booked through airline-sponsored computerized reservation systems. American Airlines reports a return on investment of 500 percent. Over the course of the years 1977 to 1986, SABRE contributed $1.5 billion to American Airlines' bottom line.

American Airlines has demonstrated a series of competitive insights, and has capitalized on them, over the years:

• The company understood and implemented new technologies that enabled SABRE to continue to expand its contribution to American Airlines. Examples include time-sharing, which dramatically improved the level of capabilities that could be offered to travel agents, and access via the Internet, to enable direct consumer ordering of tickets.

• American recognized how to leverage a process. Some analysts argue that SABRE biased travel agents toward booking American Airlines either by offering incentives to the agents or through "screen bias" by displaying American flights first (Hopper, 1990).

• The airline recognized the value of the data contained in SABRE. These data enabled American to offer frequent flyer programs and successfully manage fare wars and plane yield, ensuring that underfilled flights occurred infrequently.

• American understood the customer. SABRE has launched Travelocity, an on-line service that allows travelers to coordinate their own travel plans, from reserving and purchasing airline tickets to accessing travel and entertainment information to purchasing customized travel guides. Customers can also share travel experiences through chat groups, postings, and conferences.

• The airline understood and leveraged opportunities created when a competitive advantage had ceased to be an advantage. American eventually sold its software and expertise to competitors and others in the travel business. The company recognized that it could generate more revenue by selling its expertise and investment than by continuing to hold it within the company. For example, in 1997, American made $21.9 million by having Dollar Rent A Car Systems, Inc., and Thrifty Inc. car rentals outsource their data center and system engineering functions to SABRE.

ASAP. Another legendary example of the use of IT to improve competitive position is the Analytic Systems Automatic Purchasing (ASAP), an efficient, computerized ordering and tracking system for managing hospital supplies implemented by the American Hospital Supply Corporation (AHSC).

ASAP evolved from AHSC's efforts in the 1950s to improve hospital supply inventory control, order processing, and billing through the use of punch cards. In the 1970s, ASAP was created when these core capabilities were extended to allow hospital materials managers direct access to the ordering system by using time-sharing technology.

ASAP evolved from a focus on supply order entry and reporting to a focus on quality of service, cost management, and value-added materials management (Short and Venkatraman, 1992). A key to ASAP's success was its ability to reconceptualize business relationships. As the market shifted from a product- and price-based exchange to a value-added services approach, AHSC went beyond ordering and tracking hospital supplies and focused on customizing its system to each individual hospital. ASAP and its successors (ASAP 2, 3, 4, and 5) gave customers more power. For example, ASAP 2 allowed messages to be transmitted electronically from AHSC to sales representatives and customers. Also, ASAP 2 would automatically suggest substitutions for items that were not in stock. ASAP 3 allowed customers to build their own electronic files, using the hospital's own internal stock numbers. ASAP 4 offered minor enhancements. ASAP 5 allowed customers to place orders on their own personal computer, thereby eliminating telephone expenses (Short and Venkatraman, 1992). AHSC responded to the personal needs of its customers, adding more value to its services, by setting up teams of sales, marketing, distribution, and IT staff to analyze a hospital's ordering and receiving patterns. Like SABRE, ASAP provided market power and competitive advantage because it gave its creators access to information that their competitors could not obtain.

AHSC also gained a competitive edge by achieving status of "prime vendor of choice" among hospitals. As the prime vendor of choice, AHSC negotiates volume purchase agreements with the customer on a fixed-price basis, thus shifting purchasing decisions from price to service (Short and Venkatraman, 1992). In other words, hospitals would contract a major portion of their supplies from AHSC in return, for example, for lower inventory, reduced paper handling, guaranteed service, and fewer purchase orders. This status of prime vendor was achieved not only with ASAP but also with AHSC's broad product line. Thanks to this extensive range of products, hospitals have the advantage of "one-stop shopping" with AHSC as their supplier. Being the prime vendor of choice also helps hospitals lower administrative charges and inventory carrying costs.

Another way AHSC maintained a competitive advantage was by shifting its strategic emphasis over time. In the 1960s, ASAP was a dedicated system providing efficient nationwide distribution of hospital supplies. Now ASAP Express, designed to be the first all-vendor, all-transaction clearinghouse, is an electronic data exchange platform, similar to SABRE, where data regarding price and product availability of their competitors can be obtained. Customers can conduct business with all vendors using one system, any time of the day. Along with this strategic shift to a multivendor platform, Baxter's ValueLink program (Baxter Travenol acquired American Hospital Supply in 1985) is changing AHSC's traditional role as a distributor by assuming the role of materials manager for the hospital. This strategic partnership requires hospitals to sign a long-term contract while Baxter provides 100 percent fill rate, customized procedures, and lower inventory levels. This demonstrates the importance of shifting strategic emphasis to accommodate the evolution of traditional customer-supplier relationships.

ASAP's contribution to AHSC is impossible to overstate. ASAP can be accessed in 80 percent of U.S. hospitals. AHSC's earnings from continued operations grew from $42 million in 1974 to $237 million in 1984 (McKenney, Copeland, and Mason, 1995).

AHSC, like American Airlines, was able to leverage its core IT application competitively because it did several things very well:

• AHSC took advantage of new technologies over the years, including such things as the touch-tone phone, time-sharing, personal computers, and now the Internet, and of new technology concepts, such as electronic data interchange.

• The company evolved the system to keep pace with the needs and sophistication of its customers. What began as a means to improve the efficiency of the ordering processing for the supplies of one vendor evolved to e-mail capabilities, hospitals maintaining their own profiles, access to multiple vendors, and just-in-time supply delivery.

• It leveraged its other strengths, specifically AHSC's ability to offer a broad array of competitively priced and high-quality products and supplies.

• AHSC was able to visualize and act on significant changes in the industry— for example, health care cost pressures enabled Baxter to develop approaches to shared risk in hospital materials management—and changes in the basis of IT-centric competition—for example, expanding the narrow role of ASAP, which channeled orders only to AHSC, to that of an industry utility acting as an all-vendor-materials electronic clearinghouse.

Federal Express. The world's largest express transportation company, Federal Express (FedEx) provides an array of fast, reliable services for transporting and delivering documents, packages, and freight. The company transports time-sensitive, high-value cargo to more than 210 countries, representing more than 99 percent of the world's GDP.

A critical element of FedEx's success is the company's use of IT. Customers prefer FedEx as their express package delivery company because of IT's leverage in providing reliable, speedy service and accurate information on the status of their shipments.

FedEx's systems are used to improve the efficiency and effectiveness of internal operations by, for example, performing customer-by-customer assessment of pricing, developing earlier-in-the-day delivery options, consolidating FedEx trucking contracts, and applying the Courier Route Planner Information System, which streamlines pickup and delivery routes.

FedEx has also used IT to extend and enhance the customer's capabilities. FedEx's Powership system brings a variety of services from automated tracking, self-invoicing, stored shipping database, and report compilation and generation to the customer's desktop. Nearly two-thirds of all FedEx's volume is now processed through Powership. COSMOS is the multipurpose, multifaceted tracking system built in 1979 that connects Powership to the Digitally Assisted Dispatch System (DADS), a computer link in the courier's van. SuperTracker, which is a handheld bar-code scanner, is used by the courier to scan the package information.

Another IT enhancement of business activities is the FedEx Web site, which offers InterNetShip, which means that customers do not need to call FedEx or write out international airbills. They can print bar codes for themselves with a laser printer, arrange for a courier pickup, and then track their FedEx item. The Web site notes locations of dropoff sites, identifies easy delivery options, and provides software that customers can download like FedExShip and FedEx Tracking. FedEx continues to provide its customers with new services, like new time-of-day deliveries, new Asian routes, and instructions in different languages.

With FedEx, as in the other two cases, we see a deep understanding of the customer, an ability to capitalize on new technologies, a leverage of other strengths (in FedEx's case, it owns a package delivery system of five hundred aircraft and thirty-five thousand ground vehicles), and a continuous extension of system capabilities. Two other initiatives characterize the FedEx approach, evident also to varying degrees in the other cases:

- A radical reengineering of the business processes that surround package delivery. This successful reengineering of the organization, which spilled over to the entire industry, was achieved by recognizing IT's ability to support various process options. Furthermore, this is an example of IT strategy being developed in parallel and intertwined with business strategy, rather than IT strategy "falling out of" or being derived from the business strategy.

- A progressive transfer of control, power, and information to the customer. This transfer—for example, generating one's own shipping documents or directly determining the status of one's packages—reduced FedEx's costs and improved customer satisfaction without jeopardizing the company's core capabilities and value. On the contrary, by giving customers greater power, FedEx's value has increased.

Core Sources of Advantage

The experiences of these three companies, and those of other organizations, have led to a series of observations and conclusions, some already mentioned, about the ability of IT to provide a competitive advantage.

In most cases, IT helps organizations achieve a competitive advantage in four general ways:

- By leveraging organizational processes
- By enabling rapid and accurate provision of critical data
- By enabling product and service differentiation and, occasionally, creation
- By supporting change in organizational form or characteristics

Leveraging Organizational Processes. Information technology can be applied in efforts to improve organizational processes by making them faster, less error-prone, less expensive, more convenient, and more available (for example, allowing out-patient visits to be scheduled from home at 2 A.M.). In effect, the transaction cost of the process, from the customer's perspective, has been reduced. Examples abound:

- Automated teller machines (ATMs) have made the process of obtaining cash more convenient.
- Accounts receivable applications have made that process less expensive and faster.
- Computerized medical record systems allow more efficient accessing of information about a patient's prior encounters and treatments and less risk of overlooking relevant data.

IT leverage of processes is most effective when the processes being leveraged are critical core processes that customers use to judge the performance of the organization or that define the core business of the organization.

Patients are more likely to judge a provider organization on the basis of its ambulatory scheduling processes and billing processes than they are on its accounts payable and human resource processes. Moreover, certain attributes of these processes, and their end products, matter more than other attributes. For example, patients may judge appointment availability as more important than the organization's ability to process no-shows.

Making diagnostic and therapeutic decisions is a core provider organization process, one that is essential to its core business. Rare is the organizational process that has no bearing on or makes no contribution to organizational performance. However, certain processes are more essential to the mission of the organization and its goals than others. Customers may have limited ability to judge or evaluate these processes. For example, most patients cannot judge how well a provider organization makes diagnostic and therapeutic decisions despite the growing use and sophistication of quality measures.

Keen (1997) defines the importance of processes along two dimensions. *Worth* is a measure of the difference between the cost of a process and the revenue it generates. *Salience* is a measure of the degree to which a process is critical to an organization's identity or its effectiveness. The referral process may have high worth. The ambulatory scheduling process may be salient; it is a critical contributor to the organization's efforts to be identified as "patient-friendly." Order entry and communication may be salient because they are critical to a hospital's effectiveness.

Although provider organizations have lots of "customers"—for example, patients, providers, referring physicians, employees, and trustees—some customers matter more than others. The people who design and select information systems are not always the most important customers or have limited understanding of how customers judge the process.

IT can enable an organization to materially alter the nature of its processes. For example, the technology can enable processes or business activities to be extended over a wider geography than the immediate service area. Telemedicine enables consultation to occur with patients across the globe. The Internet can enable patients in many countries to enroll in clinical trials. IT can support an organization's efforts to franchise care operations in other states by providing access to "home" expertise.

Process can be altered or created in a manner that enables the organization to craft or significantly enhance strategic partnerships with other organizations. A process can be moved from one organization to another; outsourcing is one way to do this. For example, rather than both conducting utilization review and case management, a hospital and a managed care organization could share those responsibilities. Providers and materials suppliers have established just-in-time inventory replenishment processes. Both examples, and many others that can be imagined, are predicated on a strong IT core.

Process reexamination should accompany any effort to apply IT to process improvement. If underlying problems with processes are not remedied, the IT investment may be wasted or diluted. IT applications can result in existing processes continuing to perform poorly, only faster. Moreover, it can be harder to fix flawed processes after the application of IT since the "new" IT-supported process now has an additional source of complexity and cost to address, the "new computer system." Process reexamination, addressed thoroughly in several books (see, for example, Davenport, 1993, and Keen, 1997), can range from incremental though valuable change to more radical reengineering.

In addition to the examination and improvement of the mechanics of the process that is the target of the information system, the reexamination should question whether the process is defined correctly. Process definitions often incorporate the mechanics of the process into the core definition of the process, leading reexamination down an inappropriately narrow path. Here are two examples:

- A statement of the process such as "obtaining cash from the bank" might lead reengineering efforts to locate ATMs only at bank branches. Such ATMs might ease the burden of standing in line on a Saturday morning and hence be viewed as an improvement. However, a statement of the process as "obtaining cash" might lead analysts to consider all of the places where one needs cash— malls, theaters, airports. This might result in the placement of ATMs everywhere, leading to a far more powerful improvement in the process. A statement of the process as "buying things" might lead one to create debit cards as cash surrogates.
- A statement of the process as "obtaining a referral number" might lead to construction of an EDI link between the managed care application and the systems in the physician's office. A statement of the process as "managing referrals" might lead to abandonment of the process of obtaining referral numbers.

Recently, there has been great interest in using IT to alter the "intermediation" structures of various processes. These processes generally link a customer to a supplier.

Disintermediation would involve removing a process "middle man"—for example, selling airline tickets via the Internet, bypassing the travel agent; ordering a personal computer from the manufacturer rather than a local distributor; or specialists offering medical information on the Web, allowing patients to bypass the primary care provider.

Cementing a current intermediation role might, for example, lead a stockbrokerage to offer the ability to purchase stocks via the Internet in addition to the use of its brokers, a book distributor might support the ordering of books over the Web as a supplement to its chain of bookstores, or a mortgage firm might enable the initiation of the mortgage application in addition to providing access to its brokers.

Reintermediation involves creating a middle man where effectively, for you, there was none. The Web is being used to enable customers to find, for example, rare music recordings, specialized material for hobbies, or uncommon services. Before these offerings were available, a customer might not have had any middle man to work with.

Alteration of an intermediation structure can be effective if one reduces transaction costs, for example, by improving convenience and availability, and if one understands the process well enough not to attempt to use IT where it is inappropriate. For example, efforts to use the Web to enable a customer to perform all of the activities behind purchasing a house have had limited success because most customers want a real person to help with the complexities of the legal work and value the opinions of a real person about neighborhood schools and other subjective concerns.

Overall, the most important class of processes is coordination (Malone and Rockart, 1991; Keen, 1997). Sociologists who have studied organizational form and its effect on performance note that for the hospital, the coordination of tasks is the most critical organizational process. Coordination takes many forms:

- Communication between referring and consulting physician
- Discussion between nurses at shift change
- Propagation of managed care rules to staff in ambulatory registration and accounts receivable
- Communication between pharmacy and nursing
- Management of the operating room's schedule
- Interchanges between nursing, central transport, and the ancillary departments

Coordination involves ensuring that task performers receive the information they need to perform their jobs. This information describes the nature of the "input"—for example, the patient's problems; the desired approach to "transforming the input"—for example, the treatment plan; the desired output—for example, a consult report; and if the input has to be transferred to another task performer, the information garnered by the transferring task performer—for example, the care provided.

Enabling Rapid and Accurate Provision of Critical Data. Organizations define critical elements of their plans, operations, and environment. These elements must be monitored to ensure that the plan is working, service and care quality is high, and the environment is behaving as anticipated. Clearly, data are required to perform such monitoring.

IT can improve a competitive position by providing such data. Examples are many; here are three:

• Gathering data during registration about the patient's referring physician can help a hospital understand whether its outreach activities and market share growth strategies are working.

• Bar-code scanners at supermarkets and department stores inform product suppliers regarding which products are being purchased. This knowledge can ensure that valuable shelf space is filled with the optimal mix of product. This knowledge can also improve inventory management and allocation of manufacturing capacity. These data, when combined with data about the customer (which can be obtained when the customer presents a store card to obtain discounts), enables the store and the product manufacturer to understand the demographics of their customers, leading to more focused advertising.

- Provider order entry systems that ask for the reason or clinical indication for the procedure's being ordered not only assist the receiving department in understanding what it should do but also assist quality assurance and utilization review efforts in clarifying the dynamics of procedure utilization.

Note that *rapid* and *accurate* are relative terms. Data about product movement should be gathered and analyzed in as close to real time as possible since shelf space composition can be changed almost instantly. Analysis of physician referral patterns need not be in real time because the organization is unlikely to be able to effect a change in patterns instantly. Complete accuracy of the cost of performing laboratory tests may not be necessary because it can be clear from allocations whether a cost structure is too high or reasonable. Accuracy of the linkage between a provider and medications being ordered may be critical in order to get acceptance of any utilization analyses.

The rapid and accurate gathering of data may be the most significant and important source of a competitive advantage. Having good data about utilization may be more important than efficient ordering processes. Having good data about referring physicians may be more important than an error-free registration process. Knowing the demographics of the customers who consume your snack food, what else they buy when they buy your product, and where and when they buy may be far more important than a well-run inventory management program. Knowing who your passengers are, their fare tolerance, what time of year they fly, and their destination may be more important than managing full utilization of the aircraft.

The role of data should not imply that well-run processes are irrelevant. People would prefer to obtain services from organizations with well-run processes than from organizations that operate more loosely. Often a well-run, efficient, and convenient process may be necessary to get high-quality data. But in some cases, the process is subordinate to the need for the data. There are many examples of the competitive use of IT where the organization, accepting that its rivals will mimic process gains, focuses on the use of the data. For example, systems to support the making of an airline reservation evolved into the use of the reservation data to develop frequent flyer programs, establish mileage programs linked to credit cards, and engage in fare wars. The organizations that developed the reservation systems "sold them" to their competitors, recognizing that having such a system did not provide a sustainable process advantage.

Enabling Product and Service Differentiation. IT can be used to differentiate and customize products and services. Look at these examples:

- A financial planner offers prospective customers a Web site that helps the customers assess the savings needed to achieve financial goals such as funding college for children or having a certain income at retirement. Customers discover, after running the software, that they will be insolvent within a week after retirement. Fortunately, the financial planner is there to work with the customer to ensure that such a gloomy outcome does not occur.
- Providers establish Web sites that include information about health news, classes to reduce health risk, information on new research, and basic triage algorithms. Such information is an effort to differentiate their care from that of others.
- Supermarkets send information to customers about upcoming sales. This information is often based on knowledge of prior customer purchases. Hence a family that has purchased diapers and baby food will be treated as a household with young children. Information on sales on infant products and products directed to young parents will be sent to that household and not to households in which the purchase patterns show, for example, the regular purchase of hot dogs, snack food, and beer, indicative of a single male. The supermarket is attempting to differentiate its service by helping the household plan its purchases around "specials."

Customization and differentiation often rely on data. Effective customization presumes that we know something about the customer. Differentiation assumes that we know something about the customer's criteria for evaluating our organization so that we can differentiate our processes, products, and services in a way that is deemed to have value.

Customization and differentiation often center on organizational processes. These processes can be made unique. New processes can be created as a means of differentiation. For example, financial service firms that enable one to move one's money between money market, stock, and bond accounts create new processes that enable this movement of assets.

IT has enabled new products and services to be developed and new companies and industries to be formed. New Internet-based services and companies seem to be launched (and folded) daily. Companies that provide comparative analysis of claims and utilization data owe their existence to IT. Capitation as a scheme for financing and managing risk would be extraordinarily difficult without information technology. Several academic medical centers provide international telemedicine consultations; although it is arguable whether that is an extension of existing services or a new business.

Supporting Change in Organizational Form or Characteristics. IT can be used to improve or change certain organizational attributes or characteristics. Examples might include service quality orientation, communication, decision making, and collaboration.

- Some business and medical schools require students to own a personal computer and to do their assignments on the PC using the school's network. This emphasis is intended to accomplish several objectives, one of which is to enhance the student's comfort and skill with the technology.
- Organizations will implement groupware, for example, IBM's Lotus Notes, in an effort to foster collaboration.
- Senior management may implement a quality measurement system in an effort to encourage organizational management to be more data-driven and focused on key organizational quality parameters—in other words, "to think quality."

The value of these efforts or their impact is often unclear since the organization is often different in the end. Moreover, these characteristics tend to be quite difficult to measure at anything other than a very crude level.

Often the change in organizational characteristics is inadvertent, an unintended consequence of IT implementation. Electronic mail can be implemented to improve communication. E-mail also has the effect of speeding up decision making and altering power structures; staff will seek information from other staff, using e-mail, whom they would feel uncomfortable approaching face to face—for example, scheduling a meeting with the chief of medicine.

Sustainability of an Advantage

It is difficult to sustain an IT-enabled or IT-centric advantage. Competitors, noting the advantage, are quick to attempt to copy the application, lure away the original developers, or obtain a version of the application from a vendor who has seen a market opportunity as a result of the success of the original developers. And a sufficient number of them will be successful. Often their success may be less expensive and faster to achieve than the first organization to achieve the advantage because they learn from the mistakes of the trailblazers. A provider organization that offers its referring physicians Web access to patient results finds that its competitors will also provide such capabilities. A managed care organization that provides consumer health information and benefits management capabilities to its subscribers finds that its competitors are quite capable of doing the same.

The result can be a kind of IT arms race, a competition that provides no advantage for long and one that you must run often because the systems quickly become accepted by customers as part of basic service. No one would bank at a bank that did not offer ATM service.

In the cases discussed earlier in this chapter, the organization recognized, and perhaps knew up front, that an advantage attained at any point in time was not sustainable. Knowing that today's IT advantage is tomorrow's core capability possessed by all industry participants, the organization has several strategies that it can adopt:

• Attempt to outhustle the competition by aggressive and focused introduction of a series of enhancements to the core system that enables that system to evolve faster than the competition can and thereby maintain a lead.

• Transform the form of the advantage, as SABRE transformed the SABRE system advantage into a SABRE business advantage of generating revenues from the selling of the system and the expertise that created it to others, including competitors.

• "Freezing the system" by ceasing major investments in it and recasting the system in the role of a core production system where efficiency and reliability of operation, rather than the possession of superior capabilities, become the objectives. In this case, the organization may turn its sights to new systems that attempt to create an advantage in other ways.

• Change the basis of competition by using technology to undermine rivals' competitive strengths. Amazon.com attempts to undermine other retail booksellers' advantage of having a nationwide network of stores. This network could have been a barrier to entry; it is expensive to build hundreds of stores. Instead, Amazon.com attempts to make such a network irrelevant and possibly a liability in that the network is expensive to maintain, and overheads eat into profits.

There are ways to sustain an advantage over a prolonged period of time. In no case does a single application, by itself, result in a prolonged sustained advantage. However, an advantage can be sustained for longer than a brief period of time by leveraging some other significant organizational strength or by leveraging a well-developed, strong IT asset.

Leveraging Other Strengths. Organizations can have strengths that are quite difficult for their competitors to match (Cecil and Goldstein, 1990). Such strengths can include market share, access to capital, brand-name recognition, and proprietary know-how. IT can be used to reinforce or extend these strengths.

For example, a large integrated delivery system and a large retail pharmacy chain, both with significant market shares in a region, may decide to link the provider's medication ambulatory order entry system to the pharmacy's dispensing and medication management systems. The delivery system receives, from the pharmacy system, information as to whether the entered medication was filled, thereby improving its medical management programs. The delivery system is also able to provide a service to its patients since it can route the prescription to a pharmacy near the patient's home. The pharmacy is able to channel customers to its stores, where it believes that patients will make additional purchases when they come to pick up the medications.

The delivery system and the retail pharmacy chain find each other attractive because of their respective shares of the market. The delivery system is able to ensure significant geographical coverage for its patients filling their prescriptions. The pharmacy chain is able to ensure a large volume of customers visiting its stores. Neither party might find another party, with less market share, quite as attractive a partner. In both cases, the partnership was able to leverage an existing strength of market share.

An academic medical center that has developed, over the years, significant applied medical informatics expertise may find that such knowledge and experience enable it to develop and implement clinical information systems more efficiently and more effectively than its competitors. These systems would enable the medical center to effect IT-based improvements in the care process more rapidly than its competitors. The medical center is leveraging proprietary or scarce know-how.

A well-known academic medical center may be able to leverage its brand name and base of foreign-born physicians, who trained at the medical center, to establish a telemedicine-based international consultation service. It may also be able to leverage its brand name to improve the attractiveness of its consumer-oriented health information Web site. Consumers, confused and worried about the quality of information on the Internet, may take comfort in knowing that information is being generated by a respected source.

These advantages do not result purely from an application system or inherently from process improvement, data gathering, or service differentiation or customization. The advantages result from capitalizing on some difficult to replicate core strength of the organization through the application of IT.

Though an organization may have difficulty replicating strengths, it should be mindful that IT might be used to undermine those strengths (Christensen, 2001). For example, most integrated delivery systems have a strength of economies of scope: they offer a full range of medical services and amortize fixed costs, such as the cost of running the clinical laboratory, over this range. Under economies of scope, the incremental cost of the next medical service is small. Conversely, the incremental savings that result from eliminating a service are small.

If the country moves toward defined contributions as a means to offer health insurance, employees or patients may select their own network of providers, using a Web-based application, bypassing the network defined by the integrated delivery system. Hence the patient can select cardiology services from one IDS and oncology services from another IDS. This "cherry picking," enabled by information technology, reduces the advantages of economies of scope. Revenue from the "not picked" services becomes small, but costs have not been reduced proportionally. The IDS will face competition from organizations that focus on one service line, say, oncology. These focused service offerings may be able to obtain less expensive fixed-cost services either because they obtain them as a service, supported by IT, from a laboratory service provider, for example, or because their reduced scale of operation enables them to provide laboratory services from a lower cost base.

Leveraging the IT Asset. For most of the health care industry, the technology and applications being implemented are available to all industry participants including competitors. Any provider organization can acquire and implement systems from Eclipsys, Cerner, IDX, HBOC, or SMS. If this is true, why would a provider organization believe that it will garner an advantage from the implementation of a clinical information system from one of these vendors if a competitor can implement the same (or a similar) system—particularly if the organization has no other advantage, such as market share, that it is able to leverage with the system?

An advantage can be obtained if one, or both, of two things happen. First, one organization does a more thoughtful and more effective job than its competitors at understanding and then effecting the changes in processes or data gathering associated with the system to be implemented. The application does not provide the advantage, but the way it is implemented does. We see the difference that execution makes every day in all facets of our lives. It is the difference between a great restaurant and a mediocre one or a terrific movie and a terrible one. In neither case does the advantage derive from the idea—for example, "let's make meals and sell them"—or the fact that one executes the idea—"we've hired a cook and purchased silverware." It is the manner of execution that sets the competitors apart.

Second, if one organization is consistently able to outrun the others, it may be able to sustain an advantage. If an organization is able to develop means to implement IT faster or cheaper, it may be able to outpace its competition even if its implementations, one for one, are of no higher quality than those of its competitors. In a period of time, one organization implements four applications while the other implements three. For the same amount of capital, one organization implements five applications while the other implements three.

Such speed and efficiency can be garnered through a variety of mechanisms, none of them sufficient in and of themselves. For example, both efficiency and speed gains can be obtained through the following actions:

- Adopting and enforcing standards for technology and applications that can, for example, reduce the cost and speed up the process of developing interfaces
- Hiring and training excellent IT implementation staff
- Avoiding reflexive replacement of systems because they are "old," since system replacement diverts energy and resources
- Minimizing implementation overhead that can result from excessive dependence on committees and consensus

In general, organizations may be able to sustain an IT-based or IT-supported competitive advantage because they have an established and exceptionally strong IT asset—for example, talented IT staff, strong relationships between IT staff and the organization, and an agile technical platform (Ross, Beath, and Goodhue, 1996). This asset is able to consistently and efficiently deliver high-quality applications that enable the organization to improve its competitive position. This asset and the ways that it can provide an advantage are discussed in Chapter Three.

Technology as a Tool

IT can provide a competitive advantage. However, IT has no magic properties. In particular, the technology cannot overcome poor strategies, inadequate management, inept execution, or major organizational limitations. For example, a system that reduces the size of the nursing staff may not make the salary savings gains desired if the average nurse salary is very high or the staff is unionized. Information systems are tools. If the objectives of the building are not well understood, its design is flawed, the carpenter is unskilled, or other tools are missing, the quality of the hammer and saw is irrelevant. In the three cases described earlier, superior strategy, deep understanding of the business, the ability to execute complex transformations of the business and its core processes, and organizational ability to capitalize on their IT prowess led to the gains discussed. IT was necessary but not sufficient.

In a large number of the cases of IT use as a competitive weapon, the system leverages an existing capability of the organization (Freedman, 1991). If that capability is weak, IT may not be able to overcome the weakness. Organizations won't use, for example, a supply ordering system if the supplies are inferior in quality or too expensive or the inventory has limited scope. Recent experiences of Internet-based e-tailers highlighted the problems created by sloppy inventory management, poor understanding of customer buying behaviors such as returning purchases, or insufficient knowledge of customer price tolerance.

The referring physician won't use or value a system that provides access to hospital data if the consulting physicians at the hospital are remiss in getting their consultation notes completed and input on time or at all. High-quality, comprehensive data on care quality is diminished if the organization has limited ability or skill in improving the practice of care.

Other risks that can limit the utility of the IT tool have been documented (Cash, McFarlan, and McKenney, 1992):

• Introducing applications too early. Premature introductions may be unable to get beyond "not ready for prime time" technology and an unreceptive customer environment. Some early computerized medical record implementations have suffered this fate.

• Inadequate understanding of buying dynamics across market segments. An academic medical center that hopes its consumer-oriented Web page will lead to increased admissions may not fully comprehend the referral process if 80 percent of the organization's referrals are made by the patient's physician.

• Being too far ahead of the customers' comfort level. For example, a very large percentage of the public today is uncomfortable with the idea of personally identifiable health data being transmitted over the Internet. This discomfort has not been assuaged by the incorporation of advanced security and encryption technologies.

Finally, technology is evolving at a rapid pace, and new technologies arrive that enable new ways of supporting processes, gathering data, and differentiating and customizing products and services. In the cases reviewed earlier in this chapter, the organizations were quick to assess new technologies and thoughtful in their application. Incorporation of time-sharing and the Web are examples of new technologies that were effectively leveraged early on. This behavior suggests the following lessons:

• Organizations should have a function that scans the industry for new technologies and engages in their evaluation and experimentation.

• Critical to the assessment of new technology is the development of an understanding of the key characteristics of the technology that provide value. For example, what is it about the Web that might provide a significant improvement in organizational care delivery capabilities? (This assessment will be discussed further in Chapters Three and Four.)

• Organizations should be careful not to "fall in love" with today's technology but be able to ruthlessly jettison technology as its ability to provide a competitive distinction wanes.

Singles and Grand Slams

When we look back at organizations that have been effective at the strategic application of IT over a reasonably long time frame, we see what looks like a series of base hits punctuated by an occasional home run. One doesn't see a progression of grand slams or, in the parlance of the industry, "killer" applications (Downes and Mui, 1998).

Organizations, in the course of improving processes, differentiating services, and gathering data, carry out a series of initiatives that improve their performance. The vast majority of these initiatives don't fundamentally alter the competitive position of the organization, but in aggregate, these initiatives make a significant contribution. The difference between a great hotel and a so-so hotel is not the presence of clean sheets or hot water. Rather it is one thousand little things.

At various points in time, the organization has an insight that leads to a major leap in its application of IT to its performance. For example, airlines, having developed their initial travel reservation systems, continued to improve them. At some point, there was the organizational realization that the data, gathered by the reservation system, had enormous potency, and frequent flyer programs resulted. American Hospital Supply, having developed its supply ordering system, continued to improve it. At some point, it realized that it was in a materials management partnership with its hospital customers and not strictly in the supply ordering business.

No organization has ever delivered a series of killer or grand slam applications in rapid succession.

Organizations must develop the IT asset in such a way that they can effect the types of continuous improvements that its managers and medical staff will see possible, day in and day out. For example, in an idealized world, the organization should be able to capitalize on the improvements in ambulatory scheduling that a middle manager may see and be able to capitalize on one thousand such ideas and opportunities. The organization must also develop the "antenna" that senses an opportunity to leap and the ability to focus that enables them to effect the systems needed to make the leap. This antenna is one of the key functions of the chief information officer.

The resulting pattern may look like Figure 2.7, continuous improvement in organizational performance using IT (singles) punctuated by periodic leaps or grand slams.

It is also clear that organizations have limited ability to see more than one leap at a time. Hence planners should be careful about being too visionary or having too long a time horizon. Organizations have great difficulty understanding a world that is significantly different from the one they inhabit now or that can be only vaguely understood in the context of the next leap. We might under-

FIGURE 2.7. DEVELOPING THE IT ASSET: A SUCCESSION OF SINGLES AND GRAND SLAMS.

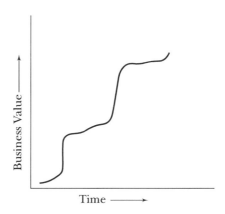

stand frequent flyer programs now, but they were not well understood, nor was their competitive value clearly recognized, at the time they were conceived. Moreover, the organizational changes required to support and capitalize on a leap can take years, at times five to seven years (McKenney, Copeland, and Mason, 1995).

Competitive Baggage

The pursuit of IT as a source of competitive advantage can result in excess baggage, which can take several forms.

Significant investment in capital, causing an increase in capital costs and in IT operating budgets (depreciation and interest), can erode margins. If several competitors are making similar investments, they may all arrive at a position where the customer sees better service or lower prices but none of the competitors has developed systems that truly differentiate one from the other, yet they have reduced their margins in the process. ATMs are an example (Lake, Mehta, Adolf, and Hammarskjold, 1998). No bank distinguishes itself because of its ATM capabilities. Customers, however, are better off. The banks must now carry the cost of operating the ATMs and funding periodic upgrades in ATM technology. Even after accounting for fees charged to banks and customers for its use, the average ATM machine has a net cost to the bank of $20,000 to $25,000. For the health care provider, investment in Web-based consumer content may have a similar outcome.

Organizations can find themselves in an IT arms race in which prudence has fled, the conversation being replaced by the innate desire to "outfeature" the competitors. The original thoughtfulness surrounding the use of IT to improve processes of care, expand market share, or reduce costs has been replaced by ego.

Governing concepts that are poorly constructed or fail to evolve can blind organizations to new opportunities. (Governing concepts are discussed in more detail in Chapters Three and Four.) For example, a concept or belief that personal computers were only for hobbyists and had no major role in a large organization, which was true in 1978, had become dead wrong by 1984. A belief that the Internet was a realm meant solely for hackers, voyeurs, and academics became wrong very quickly. Organizations often hold to beliefs and concepts long after they should be buried. This is particularly problematic when the initial belief led to an IT innovation that was very successful. People and organizations are loath to jettison beliefs that "got us where we are today." Such blindness has put companies out of business (Christensen, 1997).

Rigidity of IT can be created by poor architecture design or poor partnership selection. Many hospitals have seen, belatedly, the consequences of failure to design for application integration as they attempt to implement the integration of years of a "best of breed" strategy. The pursuit of the advantage of each department implementing the best product on the market failed to consider properties of the infrastructure (the ability to integrate applications efficiently) that would be needed to enable the organization to continue to innovate efficiently.

Organizations, overly sensitive to the IT market and grasping for an advantage, can pursue new technologies and ideas well before the utility of the idea, if any, is known. These organizations do not want to be left behind in the pursuit of the latest technology or idea for fear of ending up in the dustbin of also-rans. A very large number of ideas, technologies, and management techniques fail to live up to their initial hype. Examples include patient-focused care, total quality management, community health information networks, executive information systems, network computers, CASE tools, and client-server technology. Single-function, handheld prescription-writing devices are likely to suffer a similar fate. This should not imply that these techniques and technologies have no utility. Rather, their utility has not lived up to their press releases. (This is discussed further in Chapter Three.) The desire to achieve a competitive advantage can cause organizations to lose their senses, perspective, and at times, appropriate caution.

Extensive use of IT leads to dependence on IT. This dependence can range from staff to infrastructure performance. In several areas, such as among Web developers and network engineers, IT talent is scarce and expensive. Organizational investment in these technologies leaves them dependent on their ability to continue to attract and retain this talent. Failure to plan for this dependence can leave the organization exposed when staff turnover occurs. Similarly, organizations that have become reliant on a computerized medical record are now dependent on having a high-reliability and high-performance technical infrastructure. Tolerance of downtime evaporates. Pursuit of a competitive advantage needs to plan for the dependence that will be incurred.

Summary

IT planning has several objectives: the alignment of IT with the strategies, plans, and initiatives of the organization; the development of support for the plan; and the preparation of tactical plans. Several methodologies have emerged that improve the organization's ability to develop a comprehensive, accurate, and supportable plan. There are two forms of these methodologies: those that are derived directly from the organization's plans and strategies and those that originate from more fundamental views of organizations and competition.

IT planning is a very important organizational process. However, alignment of IT with the organization has been and remains a major challenge. The process is quite difficult. IT planning prowess cannot guarantee organizational excellence in applying IT. That excellence is significantly influenced by several factors, some of which will be discussed in Chapter Three.

IT can be very effective in supporting an organization's effort to improve its competitive position. This support generally occurs when IT is used to leverage core organizational processes, support the collection of critical data, customize or differentiate organizational products and services, and transform core organizational characteristics and capabilities.

IT is incapable of providing these advantages by itself. Its utility occurs when it is applied by intelligent and experienced managers and medical staff in the pursuit of well-conceived strategies and plans. IT cannot overcome weak leadership, inadequate strategies and plans, or inferior products or services.

The organization in pursuit of an IT-supported advantage should be careful of incurring some of the baggage that can result: reduced margins with no improvement in position, process ossification, and the irrational pursuit of mirage technologies.

CHAPTER THREE

INTERNAL IT CAPABILITIES AND CHARACTERISTICS

In Chapter Two, we discussed issues, observations, and techniques associated with aligning IT initiatives with health care organization strategies. The focus of that chapter was largely external, defining the IT initiatives necessary to respond to strategies and plans directed toward such factors as new risk arrangements, creation of a delivery system, and the activities of competitors.

In this chapter, the focus is internal to the organization. We will discuss the IT asset, which includes technology, IT staff, data, IT governance, and applications. We will also review some studies that have examined factors associated with organizational excellence in the application of IT.

This focus and these topics are critical for two reasons. First of all, IT strategic plans often call for changes in the asset in order to achieve specific organizational objectives. An objective to improve care may call for changes in applications, infrastructure, data, and IT staff. One needs asset strategies to ensure that the execution of those changes is guided by well-crafted and well-thought-out concepts. For example, what IT asset strategies will guide our efforts to establish a continuum of care? What degree of integration between applications will be required to support a continuum? Does a continuum require a common computerized medical record?

Note: Portions of this chapter originally appeared in J. Glaser, "The Siren Call of the Slogan," *Healthcare Informatics,* July 1996. © The McGraw-Hill Companies, Inc. Reprinted with permission.

Second, strategies for improving the IT asset, and the factors that have been shown to improve IT effectiveness, may be desirable in order to leverage a wide range of current and future IT plans. For example, improving infrastructure reliability may enhance the effectiveness of a series of IT initiatives. Improving the ability of the organization to prioritize IT initiatives or to evaluate initiatives may have broad organizational leverage. Enhancing the relationships between IT and the rest of the organization should advance the organization's ability to effect IT alignment and improve project execution.

Whereas strategic IT plans frame the initiatives necessary to improve organizational competitive performance, the strategies discussed in this chapter improve the ability of the IT and the organization to execute those plans. Chapter Two was, in effect, a discussion of formulation: what IT initiatives should we undertake. This chapter will discuss implementation: what IT capabilities and factors need to be in place to carry out these initiatives.

The following areas will be discussed in this chapter:

- The composition and characteristics of the IT asset, including a brief discussion of the role of the CIO
- Lessons learned and observations of the asset
- The results of studies that have examined organizational factors, including the IT asset, that contribute to highly effective use of IT; these factors will be referred to as IT-centric organizational attributes
- Achieving value from IT investments
- Factors that often influence organization choices regarding their assets, specifically, the problem of "fads" and the utility of surveys

Asset Composition and Overview

The IT asset consists of the following elements:

- *Application systems,* which are composed of the software that is used to support the work performed by organizational staff and, potentially, organizational affiliates and business partners. Examples include provider order entry, outpatient scheduling, managed care applications, and office automation.
- *Technical architecture,* which comprises the base technologies—networks, programming languages, operating systems, workstations, and so on—that form the foundation for applications and the manner in which these base technologies are put together.
- *Data,* which include all the organization's data and analyses as well as its access technologies.

- *IT staff,* the analysts, programmers, and computer operators who manage and advance IT in an organization, organization of the staff, and staff attributes—for example, is the IT function agile or unresponsive?
- *IT governance,* which consists of the organizational mechanisms (committees, policies, procedures, and work methodologies) by which IT strategies are formed, priorities are set, standards are developed, and projects are managed.

These various asset components, designed, developed, and managed under the leadership of the CIO, are the organizational IT resources that can and should be directed toward furthering organizational strategies and advancing the organization's abilities to achieve its goals. The differences between a strong asset and a weak asset can be significant. Applications that provide superior support of organizational processes are more of an asset than those that do not. IT staff who are skilled, motivated, and well organized are more of an organizational asset than staff who are not. Efficient and thoughtful procedures for prioritizing IT activities are more of an organizational asset than procedures that resemble armed conflict.

Each component contributes to the overall effectiveness of IT, and each contributes in different ways. Strategies and plans are required to ensure that the component is thoughtfully conceived, well developed, robust, sustained, and making significant contributions. IT asset strategies may look like this:

- "Due to significant environmental uncertainty, we may need to have more agile applications and infrastructure. Our agility strategy will involve creating a loosely coupled technical architecture with well-defined interfaces between layers and components."
- "We need to create a more responsive and more service-oriented IT organization. Our strategy will involve decentralizing our development and implementation teams and locating them at our affiliated hospitals."
- "We need to measure the quality and cost of our care across our delivery system. We will develop standard definitions of a small set of quality measures and create an IT department to provide analytical support for those data."

Asset Discussion

In the following sections, each IT asset component will be defined, its characteristics will be described, and a series of considerations will be presented that can be used to guide organizational definition of asset strategies.

Application Systems

Application systems are software used by the organization in the course of performing organizational activities. There are two major types of application software. Specialized application software is intended for use by a reasonably narrow set of workers performing a reasonably narrow set of tasks. Examples of specialized application software include scheduling systems, clinical laboratory systems, managed care contract analysis systems, and computerized medical record systems. General-purpose application software is intended for use by a broad set of workers or users, although the specific use can be narrow. Examples of general-purpose application software include word processing, spreadsheets, and electronic mail.

Application System Characteristics. Application systems should exhibit the following characteristics:

- They should improve existing operations and activities. Processes and activities should be more efficient and effective as a result of the implementation of application systems. Accounts receivables' days should be lower. Medication errors should be fewer. Laboratory test turnaround should be faster.
- They should provide superior support to critical processes and activities. Not all processes are created equal, nor are they equally important strategically. For processes and activities that contribute more to organizational prowess than others, the application systems support should be more than good; it should be superior.
- These systems should behave with integrity. They should perform as expected, consistently and quickly. Errors in the application software should be few or nonexistent. System performance—for example, response time—should enhance and not interfere with work.
- The application systems should have some agility. In other words, it should be reasonably efficient, effective, and timely to alter the application to respond to the needs for evolution. This response can be in the form of frequent vendor upgrades or tools that enable the organization to change the application easily and safely.
- Implementing and supporting the application should be efficient. The cost of managing the application on an ongoing basis should be modest relative to the value of the application. Application efficiency strategies can involve changing platforms to reduce support costs or standardizing an application across a delivery system in an effort to reduce application maintenance costs.

Organizations will ask themselves, "Do we have a good pharmacy system? Scheduling system? Patient care system?" To a large degree, the answer depends on how well the system fares when assessed against the characteristics just outlined.

Observations on Application Support of Processes. The characteristics of most importance are the degree to which the application enables and supports the improvement of organizational processes. In most cases, we should be able to measure the impact of the application on the organization, and that impact should serve as a rough assessment of how well this asset is performing. At times this measurement is difficult or misleading—for example, what is the measurable value of electronic mail? We also recognize that the system, by itself, does not cause improvement. The system must be properly implemented, and organizational changes may need to be made—for example, reengineering the processes to be supported by the system. Nonetheless, it is the impact on the organization that serves as the best measure of this asset component. A comparison of an application's features with those of another application or an idealized application is not an appropriate measure of application's worth unless that comparison is clearly linked to value to the organization. The evaluation of IT investments, including applications, is discussed in more detail later in this chapter.

Organizations should exercise appropriate caution when confronted with the giddiness that often occurs when new applications appear in the market or the suffocating euphoria that can surround applications with which the industry or organization lacks experience in terms of implementation, operation, or demonstrated value. The landscape is littered with examples—bedside terminals, community health information networks, executive information systems, and Internet-based health applications, among many others—with very large hype-to-value ratios. That is not to say that these applications have no value or that one cannot find settings that have happy users. However, real experiences have a way of changing euphoria to sobriety.

Organizations should look carefully, thoughtfully, and warily at the precursors or assumptions that will determine the value of major applications. Here are three examples:

• The value of executive information systems is directly related to having clear information needs on the part of senior management, senior management interest in conducting ad hoc analyses and queries with reasonably frequency, and a base of high-quality, well-integrated data. None of these precursors is inherently present in a large number of organizations.

• Enterprisewide scheduling, across a geographically dispersed delivery system, presumes that a patient (or a provider's staff) in one locality is as likely to schedule an appointment with a local specialist as to schedule an appointment with a specialist in a locality twenty miles away. This presumes that a series of factors are present: some degrees of freedom of patient movement; some knowledge, on the part of the referring provider, of the skills and existence of a wide range of specialists (and assessment that all of these specialists are of equivalent skill and deliver equivalent levels of care and service); and some exceptional rationalization of care by the IDS.

• The value of Internet-based insurance electronic data interchange is highly correlated with the ability of a provider organization's payers to receive a transaction, the degree of EDI integration with provider applications, and the ability of provider staff to act on responses received from the payer.

An existing, working application should be replaced only as a last resort. The industry appears to replace applications too frequently, often citing new technologies and application features. Of course technologies advance, as applications do, and become better over time. However, application replacement is expensive, time-consuming, and subject to opportunity costs that are often not well assessed or value gains that are insufficient. Replacement will occur, but the rationale for replacement must be very compelling. A replacement cycle that is too frequent actually retards organizational advancement because it diverts resources to areas where the gain is marginal.

Having the same application system across the enterprise has the same inherent value as having one's children dress identically. Sameness has no value per se. However, a common system can be a catalyst for developing common organizational processes and common data across the enterprise and may be necessary to consolidate a function across multiple organizations. It should be clear, however, before one pursues commonality, that the value of commonality is compelling. Developing common processes and data across several organizations is very hard work. Several IDSes have also found that the organizationwide consolidation of functions has resulted in fewer cost savings than planned, a degradation in function service performance, and a reduction in function responsiveness. This should not mean that consolidation or commonality of processes is bad. Rather it means that the rationale should be compelling and stripped of naiveté. We should remember that a common application does not de facto lead to common processes and data.

Application system strategies are varied; examples of this variety are presented in the sections that follow.

Clinical Information Systems Research and Development. Partners HealthCare has established a department within IT known as Clinical Information Systems

Research and Development (CISRD). This department is managed, and largely staffed, by individuals who have formal clinical training (physicians and nurses) and educational backgrounds in computer science. The group has several roles, three of which are related to application system strategies:

- To provide design leadership for complex clinical information systems designs, such as the entry of a structured outpatient progress note or the entry of a complex medication order
- To work with the IT Clinical Quality and Analysis department to assess the impact of clinical information systems on the care process (examples of these analyses are presented in Chapter Four)
- To provide guidance and potential answers to such questions as "How should we support the referral process?" "What should the next generation of patient-provider communication look like?" and "How should we structure clinical data?"

This department and these roles are intended to materially improve the ability of Partners' clinical information systems to improve the processes of care. The department accomplishes this goal by supporting the definition of application capabilities, identifying application features that have a significant ability to improve care, and assisting in prioritizing applications. The creation of this department was the result of a strategic conclusion that the organization's ability to have "A-plus" application support of care delivery would be materially enhanced by the existence of an applied research and development group.

Internal Development. The world is full of companies that develop applications, and a large number of them do a very good job. So how do you decide whether to buy software from them or build it yourself? The decision is subjective at times. However, several criteria guide a decision to build:

- The software one can buy isn't very good. This is more common with niche application software, for which there are few or weak competitors, than it is for software that has a large market.
- The organization's needs are unique. There are times when needs are so unique that the existing market offerings don't adequately support the work that the organization must perform. One has to be careful about claiming to be "more unique" than one really is.
- Needs are volatile or uncertain. At times an organization can be quite certain about the features that the application must possess. At other times the organization is uncertain, since it needs to garner experience with the use of the

application before it can fully understand the complete set of capabilities it will need. As this learning occurs, the organization would like to alter the application. Or the environment in which the application is being used is very volatile, and hence needs will change constantly and significantly.

• It is important to the organization that it deliver better applications than its competitors can buy. There are times when an organization's competitive performance will rest to a large degree on its having implemented an application system that is materially better than its competitors are able to implement.

• The organization needs it now. The development of an application can be (but is not always) faster to effect than the purchase of an application. Development can enable the delivery of the "crucial 30 percent" faster than the implementation of the full 100 percent.

Few delivery systems engage in significant internal development of application systems. However, improved vendor-supplied tools and advances in programming languages and techniques are enabling organizations to use internal resources to supplement or extend an application's capabilities.

The decision to engage in some level of internal development can be an outgrowth of application system strategies directed to improving application support of critical processes or enhancing application agility.

Vendor Relationships. Health care organizations have several general strategies for vendor relationships.

The organization may commit itself to a vendor's product line or engage in a "best of breed" strategy or adopt some mixture of the two—for example, all financial systems from PeopleSoft with ancillary systems purchased from niche vendors. A single vendor commitment enhances the likelihood of integration of systems and reduces the complexity of vendor management. However, the vendor's offerings may be uneven across applications, and once the commitment has been made to the vendor, organizational leverage over the vendor may decline.

Some organizations and vendors have entered into agreements in which they share business risk and reward. If the system is intended to reduce costs in the outpatient clinic, both the organization and the vendor can share in the savings. While such an arrangement may enhance vendor commitment to a successful implementation (with a broad definition of implementation) and assist in ensuring that critical system capabilities are present, such arrangements can be complex and require that the organization give the vendor some of the management responsibility formerly possessed exclusively by the organization.

These approaches to vendor relationships can be the result of application system discussions that attempt to "optimize" a complex set of trade-offs. A single-vendor approach can be more efficient and may emphasize application integration as a major contributor to support of organizational processes. A best-of-breed approach, by contrast, may accept less efficiency in order to optimize support for departmental processes. Sharing of business risk and reward with a vendor is a strategy designed to enhance the applications support of organizational processes.

Application Service Providers. An application service provider (ASP), a relatively new phenomenon, "deploys, hosts, and manages access to a packaged application to multiple parties from a centrally managed facility. The applications are delivered over networks on a subscription basis" (Le Grow and others, 2000, p. 7). Using the ASP model, a health care organization can deliver an application, such as a practice management system, without having to establish and manage the data center component of the application and hire the associated technical staff. The subscription approach enables the organization to remove the need to expend the often large amount of capital necessary to install and implement an application. Sharing the application with other organizations can mean that specific customizations to the application either cannot be made or are expensive to effect.

A decision to implement an ASP can be the result of an application system discussion that emphasizes efficiency—for example, lower up-front cost to obtain an application—and accepts some level of reasonable limitations in process support.

Application Portfolio Review. The application component of the IT asset can be evaluated as a portfolio of applications (Weill and Broadbent, 1998). An organization can array its applications across a matrix with the y-axis being a measure of "current business value" and the x-axis being an assessment of "technical quality." Each application can be plotted and given a circle. The size of the circle represents the size of the investment being made in the application, and the color of the circle represents strategic importance (see Figure 3.1). If the resulting patterns show that strategically critical applications are underfunded and of poor technical quality, the organization has a problem. If the resulting pattern shows too many applications being funded and of high technical quality but having little strategic importance, the organization has a problem.

Each application can be "valued," and the set of applications can be "valued." Portfolio review is generally done in conjunction with a discussion of IT support of organizational strategies—for example, are the organization's resources well distributed across a mixture of support for day-to-day operations and support for new, strategic initiatives? However, portfolio analysis can also lead to discussions that have broad asset ramifications—for example, a focused effort to improve application technical quality or a shift in IT project funding decisions to approve a larger proportion of strategic applications.

FIGURE 3.1. ASSESSMENT OF THE APPLICATION PORTFOLIO.

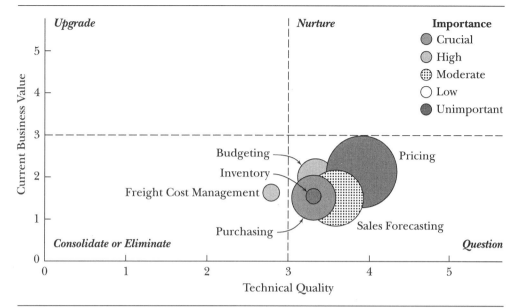

Technical Architecture

Technical architecture is often discussed by IT vendors and their customers. One hears statements such as "We use a Web-based architecture," "Our products are based on a relational database architecture." and "Our organization uses a best-of-breed architectural strategy." Statements like these confuse architecture with design. All information systems have been designed, and their design can be presented, discussed, and classified. One can talk about the location of the database in the system or the distribution of the application processing across computers or the extensibility of applications over the Internet. One can label different classes of designs with the term *architecture.* For example, applications that separate processing power between a "master" and a "slave" processor can be called a client-server architecture.

Although these classes of designs can be very important and often demonstrate insight and progress, they have no context. An organization doesn't know if Web-based or object-based "architectures," for example, are good or bad or neutral. IT professionals at times equate the column inch in the trade press or trade show decibel levels devoted to a class of designs with "goodness."

A more helpful definition of architecture is as follows: technical architecture is the set of organizational, management, and technical strategies and tactics used to ensure that platforms have critical, organizationally defined characteristics and capabilities.

There are two major types of platforms: infrastructure and clusters of applications. Infrastructure is composed of the base technologies used by an organization, such as servers and networks, and the manner in which they are put together. Clusters of applications are suites of applications that are generally viewed as being part of an integrated package—Microsoft Office, PeopleSoft financial applications, and Eclipsys clinical information systems are examples. The suites have components and are put together in specific ways.

Architecture Characteristics and Capabilities. For both types of platforms (although the remainder of this section focuses on infrastructure), an organization may decide that the critical architecture characteristics are the following.

- *Supportability.* The organization can efficiently and effectively provide day-to-day support of the infrastructure; for example, it can answer user questions, troubleshoot problems, perform backups, make minor enhancements, and run batch jobs.
- *Reliability.* The infrastructure has excellent uptime, works fast, and behaves predictably.
- *Potency.* The infrastructure uses technologies that allow the organization to buy lots of units of bandwidth, storage, and processor power for as little capital per unit as possible. Potency also means that the tools the organization has to develop applications and manage the infrastructure are powerful.
- *Agility.* The organization can replace major components of the infrastructure easily and with minimal disruption to other components. For example, the organization could change its server vendor and not have to change its server operating system or applications. At its extreme, agility would mean that an organization that wants to replace one component can ignore or need not be aware of other components. For example, an application that runs in Windows Internet Explorer may be able to ignore the workstation or a standardized transaction interface can ignore the specific technology of the receiving application. For some organizations, this may be the definition of "open systems." Agility also means that we can respond to the needs of the organization relatively rapidly and efficiently, as when adding a new remote site or adding new fields to the database.
- *Integrability.* The infrastructure eases, as much as possible, the integration of applications, data, and components of the infrastructure. Techniques such as having a common organizationwide workstation, the use of object-oriented concepts in the development of applications, the incorporation of industry messaging standards, and the implementation of a common network protocol support integrability.

Architecture capabilities are attributes of the infrastructure that can be leveraged by a wide range of applications or represent a narrow but significant addition to "what one can do." Capabilities can generally be stated with sentences beginning with "we can" or "we will be able to"—for example:

- "We will be able to provide access to radiology and pathology images from any workstation in the organization."
- "We can offer access to our clinical information systems using wireless, small-form factor devices."
- "We will be able to extend access to our systems to any part of the globe."
- "We can provide context-sensitive access to knowledge resources."

In light of the architecture's characteristics and capabilities, is the fact that an application is "Web-enabled" good or bad? It depends whether that design in general, and the application's specific implementation of it, enhances or detracts from the organization's ability to achieve the characteristics and capabilities just described. If the Web-enabled application uses a database management system that is different from the organizational standard and hence reduces the ability to integrate the application with other applications, being Web-enabled can be bad. If the application, despite being Web-enabled, is unstable, it is bad. If being Web-enabled means that the application can be accessed from anywhere on the globe, it could be good. If the application conforms to the standards, is highly reliable, and uses commodity technology—for example, Intel-class machines—that enhances its potency, it may be good.

Other statements of the goals of architecture have been developed. For example, Weill and Broadbent (1998) note that the goals of an architecture are to enable an enterprisewide infrastructure to achieve compatibility between various systems, specify the policies and mechanics for delivering the information technology strategy, describe the technological model of the organization, cut through the multivendor chaos, and move toward vendor independence.

Technical Architecture Strategies. Architectural strategies are composed of four major elements. The first element is statements of desired characteristics that are clear and, where possible, measurable. What does agility or supportability mean to us? How would we know if reliability or supportability has been improved? Could we measure it? The statements should be robust; in other words, the statement will endure as the specific products change and evolve. For example, an organization's definition of supportability should survive the industry's movement from Windows 95 to Windows 2000. The changes in products should enhance the ability of the organization to realize the desired characteristics, but the definition of the characteristics doesn't change.

The second element is statements of desired capabilities that are clear. To how much of the globe do we want to provide access, and is this access to all of our applications or some of them? Does image access need to provide diagnostic-quality images or not? Capability statements should also have an associated statement of value. Why would one want to invest the time and energy to provide these capabilities? How will patient care or administrative effectiveness be improved?

The third element is the statement of specific components, such as Cisco routers, or classes of components, such as source routing, that will form the building blocks of the architecture. These components have features that enable them to be more reliable, supportable, and so on. As the organization upgrades its components or shifts to new components, it should understand how each change enhances its ability to improve characteristics or capabilities. This is particularly true when the change is expensive and possibly disruptive. For example, how does Windows 2000 enhance supportability or reliability? What important capabilities will handheld devices provide?

The fourth element is the approaches to putting together or fitting the components such that the whole achieves the desired characteristics and delivers the desired capabilities. One can engineer a very unreliable network or a very reliable one. One can engineer a network such that the movement of images cripples the performance of other applications or is not noticeable by the users of the other applications. The same components may also be engineered to arrive at different designs such that the resulting system is Web-enabled or not.

The approaches to fitting can be very diverse; for example:

- The organization can standardize on a workstation (or database or development language) to enhance supportability.
- Fault tolerance, disk mirroring, and rigorous application testing methodologies can all improve reliability.
- Internal development of applications, standardized interfaces, and the selection of market-standard operating systems can all enhance agility.
- The choice of commodity technologies or an aggressive technology replacement cycle—for example, 40 percent of the workstations are replaced every year—can improve potency.
- Network segmentation can enable image movement.
- A virtual private network service or the Internet can provide some forms of global access.

The approaches for fitting run the gamut from choices of technology to adoption of standards to engineering of component relationships to staff support mechanisms to technology obsolescence tactics to organizational policies regarding technology heterogeneity.

Changes in Characteristic and Capability Importance. The importance of architectural characteristics and capabilities can change or vary.

Importance can be influenced by "today's issues." If an organization has significant reliability problems, that attribute will be viewed, appropriately, as deserving the full attention of IT management even if that attention detracts from efforts to improve agility.

The rate of business change and technology change will also influence the importance of these attributes (GartnerGroup, 1998a). If the technology is to support volatile and critical business activities, agility is paramount.

Importance can be influenced by the nature of organizational work. If the technology is to support core transaction activities that are used directly by customers, as in the case of airline reservations, then reliability and supportability become paramount.

In general, when the nature of an organization's business seems to be on the edge of significant change, the technical architecture should be examined to see if the relative importance of characteristics and capabilities needs to change. For example, organizational efforts to expand the service area or focus heavily on improving care quality can increase the emphasis on extensibility of applications and reliability, respectively.

Technology change is generally continuous and accelerating. However, the technology change that matters to an organization is the change that surrounds the technologies that it is using or intends to use. An organization may see little relevant technology change in some segments despite sweeping changes in the technology industry.

Component choices and fit approaches will also change as new technologies and techniques enable the organization to consider new architectural strategies. The Web, component-based architectures and high-performance, high-availability servers are examples of such technologies. New technologies often present characteristic trade-offs—for example, agility may be improved, but reliability is a problem—and capability trade-offs—for example, providing global access may hinder the development of a highly secure environment.

Though the choices, fit approaches, and relative importance of characteristics and capabilities will change, the definitions of technology architecture characteristics and capabilities adopted by an organization tend to be static for long periods of time.

Architecture Representation. There is utility to expressing architecture in terms that a nontechnical audience can understand, as during the budget development process. Doing so is generally easier for application architectures than for technical architectures.

Application architectures can be well presented by diagrams of components and their interrelationships and by narrative descriptions of workflow. Figure 3.2 depicts the components for Partners HealthCare's clinical information systems. Exhibit 3.1 presents a paragraph from a narrative description of clinical information systems workflow as an illustration of fit.

FIGURE 3.2. COMPONENTS FOR PARTNERS HEALTHCARE'S CLINICAL INFORMATION SYSTEMS.

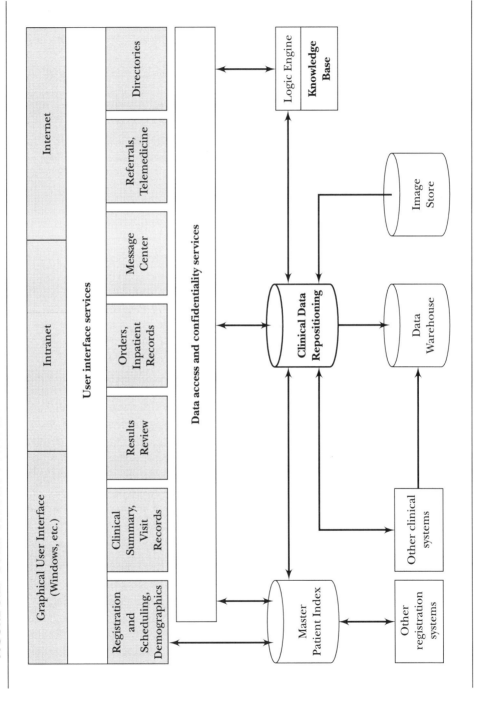

EXHIBIT 3.1. NARRATIVE DESCRIPTION OF CLINICAL INFORMATION SYSTEMS WORKFLOW.

Dr. Smith is a primary care physician at a community practice outside of Route 128. She has a workstation at her desk, connected to the Partners network. She arrives at her practice on a weekday morning, ready for a full day of primary patient care. Upon arriving at her desk, she checks her workstation and finds several items waiting in its electronic in-box.

The computer first reports on the status of the two patients in Dr. Smith's practice who are currently hospitalized. The report shows the narrative status and current plan for each, as well as a summary of the patient's most recent test results, medications, and procedures. The screen also displays the phone number of the patient's floor, as well as the name and beeper of the inpatient physician. By selecting a button, Dr. Smith can page the doctor, call the nurse on the floor, or leave electronic mail.

The in-box also indicates that there is news about two of the five patients who are in active consultation referral. One, sent to an orthopedist, has had an MRI; the results are available by selecting a view button. Another, sent for neurology consultation, has finished the consultation; the screen displays the summary report.

Dr. Smith next proceeds to the Results Manager section of the in-box. It shows her all new results of tests and diagnostics studies on her patients. Dr. Smith selects the first patient and notes a normal mammography result. Choosing from the available options, she opts to send a letter to the patient, informing her of the result. The computer automatically updates the patient's health maintenance profile.

Drazen and Metzger (1998) present well-developed and thoughtful descriptions of the application architecture to support enterprisewide processes for an IDS.

Representing technical architecture is more difficult. At times organizational leadership will be presented with a diagram that shows multiple boxes, some squiggly lines, and an oval or two. The diagram may be a significant reduction of a large drawing onto an $8\frac{1}{2}$-by-11-inch sheet of paper, making the whole thing illegible. It might be titled "Our Technical Architecture" or "Current Systems Environment." Figure 3.3 presents a typical architecture diagram for a hospital information system. Or an organization might see an oval that has lines from it to boxes with labels indicating applications and organizations. Figure 3.4 presents a typical architecture diagram for an IDS system.

FIGURE 3.3. TYPICAL HOSPITAL INFORMATION SYSTEM ARCHITECTURE DIAGRAM.

CURRENT SYSTEMS ENVIRONMENT

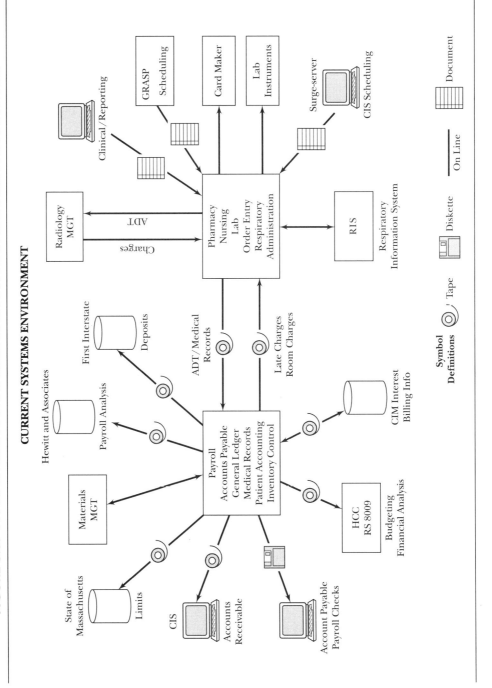

FIGURE 3.4. TYPICAL INTEGRATED DELIVERY SYSTEM ARCHITECTURE DIAGRAM.

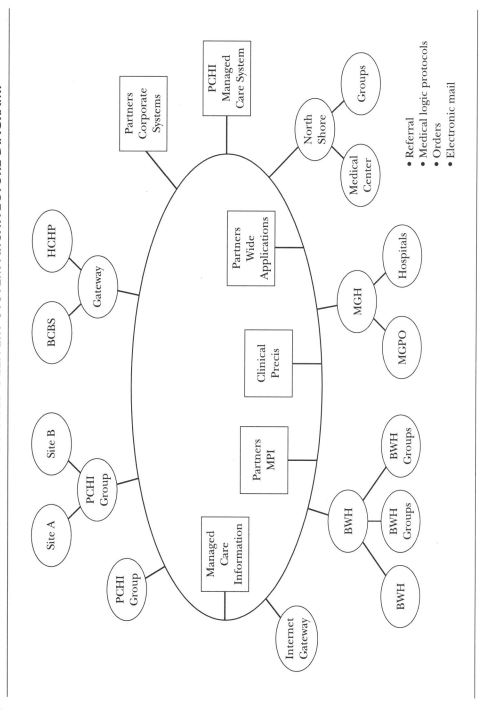

Such diagrams may help organizational leaders understand some of the concepts behind the architecture. However, architectures are strategies and tactics to achieve goals; they are not diagrams. This paragraph is not intended to denigrate the utility of such diagrams but rather to ensure that we, who put them up on the overhead projector, remember that these diagrams, in and of themselves, are insufficient statements of architecture.

Three examples of technical architecture strategy are discussed in the paragraphs that follow: the Partners technical strategy function, Partners' selection of an application platform, and considerations in the design of wireless applications.

Technology Strategy Function. A technology strategy function was established at Partners. The function has several objectives:

- To define the Partners technology architecture
- To identify technologies that materially advance both the ability of IT to support Partners' strategies and plans and the efficiency and effectiveness of IT execution and operations
- To define the experimentation or data gathering activities necessary to determine whether a particular new technology is capable of supporting the stated objectives
- To define the IT groups, teams, or industry partnerships necessary to design, develop, and implement critical technologies
- To develop mechanisms to document and communicate the Partners technology strategy, direction, and architecture

This function is overseen by the Technology Strategy Committee. Committee membership includes the leaders of core technology groups within Partners (application development, medical imaging, operations, network engineering and support, server management, and telecommunications) and Partners' IT leadership (hospital CIOs and the Partners CIO).

The committee is staffed and chaired by the technology planning department, which has the task of developing committee agendas and ensuring that the decisions of the committee are carried out.

Major agenda items for the committee in 2001, for example, were implementation plans for Windows 2000, determination of the role and the technology to support wireless computing, and directory and security services.

The technology strategy function is an outgrowth of a strategy discussion on technical architecture, specifically, the need to create an ongoing mechanism for architecture strategy development.

Application Platform. Partners bases its clinical information systems on Intersystems Cache, an application platform. Cache includes a development language, a database management system, and operating system capabilities needed to manage large-scale process interoperability. This choice (not meant to imply an endorsement of the product) illustrates the refinement of several infrastructure characteristics and serves as an example of mapping characteristics to specific features of a technology. XML objects, for example, are a technology feature that can support integrability and agility.

The platform, when engineered in conjunction with network and server technologies, is able to provide very high availability (reliability). If a process loses a connection to a server, it will automatically attempt to establish another connection through another path.

Cache has been integrated with Web services, Win 9X/Visual Basic, Oracle and SQL Server, PDAs, and HIPAA-compliant EDI. In addition, Cache programs have been wrapped to appear as Java, Com, and XML objects (integrability).

The platform has been scaled to respond to very large transaction processing demands; for example, it performs an average of 10.7 billion cross-platform reads and writes of programs and data every day. Applications, based on the platform, can be delivered to small sites, such as the office of a solo practitioner, and large sites, such as a nine-hundred-bed academic medical center (agility).

The Cache platform was chosen for its ability to meet a set of infrastructure characteristics.

Wireless Considerations. Partners, like many health care organizations, is in the early stages of deploying wireless applications such as medication administration record, medication ordering, and results retrieval systems. Effective deployment of wireless applications requires that the infrastructure possess many of the characteristics that have been discussed in this section. The following paragraphs are excerpted from internal Partners documents (Flammini, 2001) and illustrate the detailed application of the principles of infrastructure characteristics.

Browser-Based Presentation Layer

Wireless devices are now equipped with Web browsers. The browsing capabilities vary among handheld platforms but are adequate and improving.
   • A browser-based wireless environment allows for a high degree of device independence. With a browser presentation layer, application middleware services generate Web pages for the user presentation without too much regard for the specific operating system environment on the wireless client. As winners and losers emerge in the wireless handheld marketplace and as new wireless

devices appear, Partners can move adroitly to new wireless platforms without significantly rearchitecting its applications. (agility)

• The presence of a Web browser on the wireless client obviates the need for a complex software distribution scheme because applications are network-resident. Clients access Web URLs for application functionality, and software changes are made "server-side."(supportability)

• The operating system for the Microsoft Pocket PC platform (CE 3.0 and Pocket IE 3.0, respectively) are now reasonably potent. In cases where browser capability is more critical, we prefer to use the Microsoft OS browser architecture. The Palm OS/Web Clipping browser, while adequate for the simplest HTML commands, is much more limited. (potency)

Robust, Reusable Middleware Layer

For several years, Partners has developed multitier applications (client-server and Web), resulting in the creation of a "middleware services" layer.

• This collection of stateless service objects exposes underlying business logic in a platform-neutral manner. Some examples: role-based authentication, query and retrieval of patient data objects (active medications, problem list, allergies, lab results), decision support rules, and master patient index lookups. (agility, integrability)

• Increasingly, these services have become XML-based, with an emphasis on delivering content to a device-independent setting, in other words, the separation of content and presentation. This fits nicely into a wireless strategy, because middleware services can deliver content to a Web server, where the content can be wrapped with HTML or XSL for presentation, and then passed back to the wireless browser client. This method of delivering content results in a fairly modest amount of new development while preserving investment in existing services. (agility, integrability)

Data

The data component of the IT asset is composed of the following:

• Data recorded on some medium
• Organizationally defined data coding conventions, standards, and definitions, such as ICD-9 codes, ZIP codes, and standards for identifying whether a physician is a primary care provider or not
• Policies, procedures, and management mechanisms that guide the capture, "cleaning," and use of data

- Technologies that capture, store, and support the access and analysis of data—for example, database management systems and reporting packages

Data Characteristics. Organizational data have five critical characteristics:

- They must be accurate. Data that are accurate capture, with tolerable error, the "true" state of some phenomenon, activity, or thing. If the data say that 24 percent of a provider organization's patients are subscribers of one HMO, that should be a fair reflection of the truth.
- They must be timely. The interval between the time or period when someone wants to make a decision or check the status of an activity and the time of the availability of the data should be short relative to factors such as the pace of change, the organization's ability to move with a certain speed, and the urgency of dependent decisions.
- They must be easily understood. Data should have a definition that is consistent and comprehensively understood by all users of those data. An "encounter," for example, should have a common definition throughout the enterprise.
- They must be accessible. Decision makers should be able to access, with minimal difficulty, the data they need to make decisions and monitor activities.
- They must be efficient. The capture, transformation, and reporting of data should be efficient.

These desired characteristics are not particularly controversial. One can develop other characteristics, but no one would dispute the usefulness of accurate, timely, well-understood, accessible, and efficiently gathered data.

Despite this consensus, the quality of data in most organizations is often relatively poor. The major contribution of executive information systems and decision support systems, all the rage several years ago, was for most organizations to point out the exceptionally poor quality of organizational data. Executives found that they were able to bring forth, with the touch of a button, multicolored graphs of garbage.

Data, as discussed in Chapter Two, can be a very important source of competitive advantage and critical for organizational monitoring of its performance and strategic progress. Data may be the most unforgiving component of the IT asset. If the organization implements lousy application systems or unreliable technologies, it can replace them. If the organization hires someone who is incompetent, it can remove the person. But if the organization allows poor-quality data to enter into its systems or develops an ill-conceived coding scheme, it may not be able to correct the problem.

Data Strategies. There are four major areas where strategies regarding data are necessary. The first is the definition of what data to collect. This is a complicated matter; the answer depends to a very large extent on organizational definitions of strategy, critical success factors, key environmental variables, and essential performance areas. Data can be gathered to assess market share, financial performance, care outcomes, cost of care, conformance of care to protocols, appointment availability, and patient satisfaction. All of these areas, and others, involve discussions of specific data elements, data definitions, sources of data, acceptable data error rates, users of data, and confidentiality of data.

The second area involves the definition of which data should be standardized throughout the enterprise and which standards should be used. In some areas, the standardization choices are constrained; for example, general accounting practices have a significant influence on the definition of data on financial performance. In other areas, a small number of choices exist, but the choices have quite different ramifications and limitations, as is the case for schemes for coding patient problems. And in some areas, the organization may have great latitude, as in the definition of market share, although the choices, again, have very different ramifications.

The third area is the identification of data management and access technologies. Technologies and techniques are varied, and the industry is often awash in discussions on data management technologies. The air is full of new buzzwords and trendy terms such as data mining, data warehouses, data marts, OLAP (on-line analytical processing) tools, and operational data stores (Marietti, 1998; GartnerGroup, 1998b). Despite the frenzied trendiness, these techniques and technologies do have important distinctions and contributions.

The fourth area is the development of organizational mechanisms and functions to manage data and perform activities designed to improve the characteristics of the data component of the IT asset. These mechanisms are often decentralized; for example, Finance manages data on financial performance, Marketing may manage data on market share and patient satisfaction, Health Information Management is responsible for coding of procedure and disease data, and Quality Assurance may manage data on outcomes.

Regardless of the responsibility distribution, organizational leaders should recognize that developing and maintaining high-quality data requires all of the following (Glaser and Williams-Ashman, 1990):

• Staff who are responsible for managing data quality. These staff document data meaning and ensure data integrity by developing and enforcing data management techniques such as data dictionaries and initial and retrospective data entry checks and edits and by supporting "official databases." Responsibility means that their job descriptions are explicit about these tasks. These staff can be asked to oversee data generated externally and used by the organization.

• Senior management support. Data quality involves changes in applications and work processes and budgets to support the data quality and management function. Data quality often requires that those who enter data undertake additional work for the benefit of someone else who is "downstream." Ensuring high-quality registration data may offer little immediate advantage to the registration clerk but is terribly important to the accounts receivable clerk.

• A recognition that whereas technology can be sexy; managing data quality is generally not. Trying to determine how an organization managed to perform a hysterectomy on a twenty-year-old male, as the data indicate, requires the skills of a good detective and often involves the drudgery of a stakeout. This work is not always exciting. Nonetheless, sexiness has never been a good predictor of importance.

Data management should also include developing, maintaining, and making widely available the inventory of data resources and specifying the terms and conditions under which one organizational unit may have access to another's data (Levitin and Redman, 1998).

Two examples of data strategies are presented in the sections that follow. The first discusses the creation of clinical quality analysis capabilities, and the second briefly examines knowledge management.

IDS Quality Measurement. The creation of an IDS-wide function to measure care quality and patterns would be an example of a data IT asset strategy. Such a function would establish a database that contains a superset of quality data and metrics used by individual organizations within the IDS. The function would generate IDS-wide reports and analyses based on these data.

This function would need to be guided by an overall steering committee, composed of medical staff leaders and senior quality management staff, that developed policies and procedures governing the use of data and defining areas of focus for quality improvement efforts. This committee could be supplemented by a working group that developed specific data definitions and resolved methodological issues, such as means to stratify data to reflect patient acuity. These groups would complement and support organization-specific quality measurement efforts.

Figure 3.5 provides an overview of a proposed quality management function at Partners HealthCare. The Partners Care Analysis Committee (PCAC) serves as the overall steering committee. The Quality Management Group (QMG) is the working group. These committees, and the Partners Clinical Data Warehouse, support quality measurement and reporting activities at the Massachusetts General Hospital (MGH) and the Brigham and Women's Hospital (BWH).

FIGURE 3.5. PROPOSED QUALITY MANAGEMENT ORGANIZATION STRUCTURE FOR PARTNERS HEALTHCARE SYSTEMS.

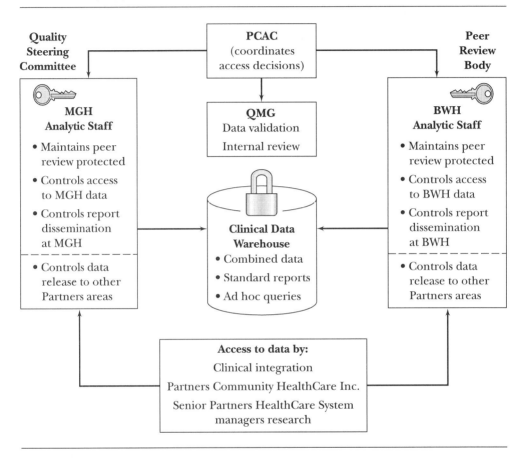

The data strategy discussion involves the formation of groups such as these and the definition of their responsibilities and activities.

Knowledge Management. Under the IT asset taxonomy, knowledge management would be considered a form of data. Proponents would argue, correctly, that knowledge management is different in character and complexity than managing data as an asset, although the two areas overlap. Nonetheless, the areas covered by the development of a knowledge management strategy and the steps taken would be similar to those covered by a data asset strategy discussion. (See Davenport and Prusak, 1998, for a thorough discussion of knowledge management.)

For example, a provider organization faces several knowledge management challenges:

- Defining appropriate medication use in specific clinical situations
- Disseminating managed care contract provisions
- Translating clinical research to practice
- Training health care professionals

In a knowledge management undertaking, the organization may decide to improve its management of knowledge regarding disease management. The organization would identify those diseases, because of prevalence or cost, that would become the targets of disease management. An organizational effort could be undertaken to standardize protocols and guidelines for cancer screening, health maintenance, and treatment of lower back pain, asthma, hypertension, and depression. Web technologies could be employed to provide access to protocols and guidelines, and health maintenance reminders could be built into computerized medical record systems. Committees of providers would need to be formed to provide ongoing management and revision of disease management guidelines and protocols.

IT Staff

The staff component of the IT asset has three major aspects:

- Attributes of the staff
- Core staff capabilities and competencies
- Organization of the staff

Staff Attributes. High-performing IT staff have several general characteristics in common:

- They execute well. They deliver applications, infrastructure, and services that display a sound understanding of organization needs. These deliverables occur on time and on budget and earn high marks for professional comportment from others involved in the project.
- They are good consultants. They advise organizational members on the best approach to the application of IT given the organizational problem or opportunity. They advise when IT may be inappropriate or the least important component of the solution. This advice ranges from help desk support to systems analyses to new technology recommendations to advice on the suitability of IT in furthering an aspect of organizational strategy.

• They provide world-class support. Information systems require daily care and feeding and problem identification and correction. This support needs to be exceptionally efficient and effective.

• They stay current with their expertise, keeping up-to-date on new techniques and technologies that improve the ability of the organization to apply IT effectively.

A wide variety of techniques can assist IT management in their efforts to improve staff attributes—for example, the ability of staff to manage projects and to ensure that staff are current in their expertise.

We shall look at two major strategic issues regarding staff attributes. The first involves the attraction and retention of staff. The market for talented and experienced IT staff will be competitive for some time (National Research Council, 2001).

Recruitment and retention strategies involve making choices about the work factors and management practices that will be changed and how they will be changed in order to improve the ability to recruit and retain staff. For example, should the focus be on salaries or career development or physical surroundings or some combination of these factors?

For example, Partners IT managers were asked to identify the factors that make an organization a great place to work and then rated Partners IT against those factors. The factors identified by the managers were the following:

• Salary and benefits
• The physical quality of the work setting, for example, well-maintained surroundings
• The caliber of IT management
• The amount of interesting work
• The importance of the mission of the organization
• Opportunities for career growth
• The adequacy of communication about topics ranging from strategy to project status
• The reputation of the overall organization and IT

The results of the managers' ratings of Partners IT against these factors are presented in Table 3.1.

On the basis of these scores, Partners IT leaders decided to focus on the following improvements:

• Establishing more thorough and better-defined career paths and development programs for all staff

TABLE 3.1. PARTNERS HEALTHCARE IT MANAGERS' RATINGS OF "GREAT PLACES TO WORK" FACTORS.

Factor	A	B	C	D	F
Compensation and benefits	1	14	12	3	0
Work environment	4	17	4	3	2
Good management	6	13	8	3	0
Interesting work	12	2	0	0	0
Mission	17	12	1	0	0
Career growth	4	19	5	0	2
Communication	0	8	15	2	5
Status of organization	0	17	10	3	0
Total	61	95	48	11	9

Note: A through F are letter grades awarded by thirty IT managers. The numbers indicate how many of the thirty IT managers awarded each letter grade for each factor.

- Improving training opportunities, ranging from brown bag lunches with invited speakers to technical training to supervisory training to leadership training
- Reviewing work environment factors such as parking, free amenities such as soda, and office furniture
- Improving communication through mechanisms such as a monthly e-mail from the CIO, videotaping staff meetings for access through streaming media, and regular dinners and lunches hosted by the CIO and deputy CIO

These steps are important. Fundamentally, people like to work where the job is challenging and meaningful. They prefer places where they like their co-workers and respect their leaders. They stay in jobs longer when they are proud of the organization, its mission, and its successes.

A second strategic issue surrounds the ability of outsourcing or task sourcing to obtain needed expertise and experience. Outsourcing can also be a strategy to address issues of core staff capabilities and competencies (discussed in the next section).

Experiences with full outsourcing have been mixed (Strassmann, 1997), with a significant number failing to deliver expected cost reductions and service improvements. Partial outsourcing or task sourcing of such things as deployment of workstations or HIPAA compliance work appears to be more effective. These partial outsourcing arrangements enable organizations to obtain expertise and competencies that may not be viewed as core organizational competencies (although necessary competencies), address temporary staff needs, or obtain staff that the organization cannot afford or is unable to hire. Lacity and Willcocks (1998) provide an overview of strategies that enhance the effectiveness of IT sourcing.

Examples of such practices include selective rather than total outsourcing, sourcing decisions jointly made by IT managers and senior leaders, and inviting internal IT bids for the "sourcing business."

Core Capabilities and Competencies. IT staff who execute well and provide excellent consulting and other support are very important. However, organizations should identify a small number of areas that constitute core IT capabilities and competencies. These are areas where getting an "A-plus" matters. The strategic question involves the definition of these core capabilities and the development of plans to establish A-plus competencies.

For example, in 1998, Partners HealthCare System defined three areas of core capabilities; base support and services, care improvement, and technical infrastructure.

Base Support and Services. This category of core capabilities included three subcategories:

- Operational management and support of a high-performance technical infrastructure
- Front-line support, for example, PC problem resolution
- Project management skills

While skills in these areas are probably always very important, they reflect a particular emphasis, across all Partners' centralized services in 1998, for example, Finance and Human Resources, on improving service quality. These departments had seen their service suffer as a result of their efforts to integrate their functions across the organizations in the delivery system. Restoring the groups to prior levels of service, and exceeding prior levels, was judged to be a critical Partners strategic emphasis.

Care Improvement. Central to the Partners agenda was the application of IT to improve the process of care. (A series of strategies surrounding this emphasis are discussed in more detail in Chapter Four.) One consequence was to establish, as a core IT capability, the set of skills and people necessary to apply IT innovatively to medical care improvement. An applied Medical Informatics function was established to oversee a research and development agenda. (This function was discussed earlier in this chapter as an application system strategy.) Staff skilled in clinical information systems application development were hired. A group of experienced clinical information system implementers was established. An IT unit of health services researchers was formed to analyze deficiencies in care processes, identify

IT solutions that would reduce or eliminate these deficiencies, and assess the impact of clinical information systems on care improvement. Organizational units, possessing unique technical and clinical knowledge in radiology imaging systems and telemedicine, were also created.

Technical Infrastructure. Recognizing the critical role played by having a properly conceived, executed, and supported technical architecture, infrastructure architecture and design continued to serve as a core competency. The technology strategy function discussed earlier in this chapter was created. Significant attention was paid to ensuring that extremely talented architectural and engineering talent was hired along with staff with terrific support skills.

IT Organization. There are three aspects of the IT organization for which strategies must be developed:

- The definition and formation of departments or major functions
- The form of the IT structure (for example, matrixed or flat)
- Attributes of the IT organization as a whole (for example, agility)

There are multiple considerations in defining the departments or major functions within an IT organization, which may include financial application implementation and support, telecommunications, telemedicine, and decision support. One of the primary strategic considerations is the "organizing unit or concept."

One can organize around any of the following:

- Sites or members of the IDS—for example, dedicated IT staff to support each organizational member of the IDS with a site CIO
- Infrastructure and platform support—for example, a unit of staff responsible for implementing and supporting the IDS network or a specific platform, such as the mainframe
- Applications or application suites—for example, financial systems or patient care systems
- Processes—for example, a unit of IT staff responsible for systems support for all outpatient scheduling and registration activities across the IDS
- Classes of care—for example, inpatient, subacute and primary care
- IT research and development—for example, the investigation of new technologies

An IT organization is likely to organize around more than one concept; for example, it may have site IT organization staff and CIOs and central support of some platforms. And an IT organization is unlikely to try and adopt all of the concepts because some form of dysfunction or even chaos would quickly follow.

The IT organization should organize in a manner that mirrors the overall organization of the IDS. The IT organization should adopt the organizing concepts of the IDS, and the IT organization should be a reflection of the IDS. For example, if the IDS has CEOs for each member hospital, the IT organization should have organization CIOs. If the IDS has centralized finance, the IT organization should have a function responsible for systems support of finance.

The strategic questions in determining the major IT departments are which concepts will be used in defining departments, whether the departments represent clearly circumscribed clusters of like expertise or common goals, and whether the resulting set of departments is comprehensive in scope.

The form of the IT organizations in an IDS are invariably matrixed. Kilbridge and Drazen (1998), in a study of IDS IT organizations, found three dimensions that defined the matrix. The functional dimension was devoted to IDS-wide infrastructure—for example, communications network and enterprise master person index—and the support of IDS-wide consolidated functions, such as finance. The geographical dimension was devoted to supporting distinct geographical sites or logically separate provider sites, such as one of the IDS community hospitals. The cross-continuum process-oriented dimension might support acute care in general or a "carve-out" such as oncology services. Figure 3.6 depicts a two-dimensional structure based on function and geography. Figure 3.7 shows a two-dimensional structure based on function and process.

FIGURE 3.6. TWO-DIMENSIONAL ORGANIZATIONAL STRUCTURE BASED ON FUNCTION AND GEOGRAPHY.

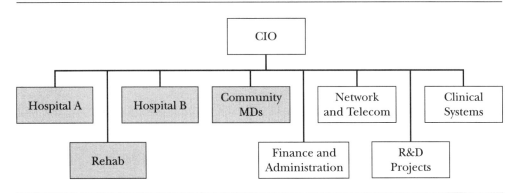

Source: P. Kilbridge and E. Drazen, "Information Systems for IDNs: Best Practices and Key Success Factors," *Proceedings of the 1998 Annual HIMSS Conference* (Chicago: Healthcare Information and Management Systems Society, 1998). Reprinted with permission.

FIGURE 3.7. TWO-DIMENSIONAL ORGANIZATIONAL STRUCTURE BASED ON FUNCTION AND PROCESS.

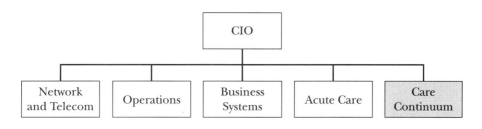

Source: P. Kilbridge and E. Drazen, "Information Systems for IDNs: Best Practices and Key Success Factors," *Proceedings of the 1998 Annual HIMSS Conference* (Chicago: Healthcare Information and Management Systems Society, 1998). Reprinted with permission.

The matrix form of IT is largely a reflection of the matrix structures of most IDSes. IDSes have evolved some form of central control and functions and local autonomy. The degree of centralization may vary, but it is unusual to find a pure hierarchy in an IDS or an IDS with no central management.

There is no single way to organize. IDSes will differ in their efforts to consolidate some functions and not others. IDSes will vary in their efforts to create "lines of business," for example, diabetes care or women's health, which cut across its member organizations. And most organizations experiment, over time, with changes in the degree to which they centralize and decentralize as they discover the limitations of the current structure and forget about the limitations of prior structures.

The strategic discussion surrounds the selection of organizational form and the reasons for selecting it and ensuring that the resulting form is an adequate mirror of the overall form of the organization.

IT organizations, like people, have characters or attributes. They can be agile or ossified. They can be risk-tolerant or risk-averse. The characteristics can be stated, and strategies to achieve desired characteristics can be defined and implemented. Although organizations can have any number of characteristics, we will briefly discuss two: agility and innovativeness. These two are illustrative of any organizational characteristic and are generally viewed as desirable.

An agile organization would probably have several attributes that could include the following:

- The ability to form teams quickly. This implies some level of "slack" in resources and the ability to "park" initiatives, currently in progress, as members of that initiative are included in the new team.

- Appropriate "chunking" of initiatives such that there are multiple points, along the initiative, during which the project could be stopped and still deliver value in its stopped state. For example, the rollout of a computerized medical record, which may call for ten clinics per year, could be stopped temporarily at four and still deliver value to those four.
- Decision-making forums, such as IT steering committees, that are able to make decisions and encumber resources quickly.

An organization that emphasizes agility will also attempt to create agile platforms; for example, it will select and implement applications that have potent tools that enable the organization to enhance the applications rapidly. It would also try to create loosely coupled architectures, for example, architectures that provide efficient and standard interfaces between applications and enable applications to be replaced without causing significant changes in other applications (almost "plug and play").

An organization that is innovative could have characteristics such as these:

- Reward systems that encourage new ideas and successful implementation of innovative technologies and applications
- Punishment systems that are loath to "punish" those involved in experiments that failed
- Small "grants" that can be obtained outside of the normal budget process to fund the pursuit of interesting ideas
- Dedicated research and development groups within IT

The foregoing discussion of organizational characteristics does not cover all characteristics, for example, a service-oriented IT organization. Moreover, ample literature exists on the topic of molding and creating organizational cultures that have desired characteristics.

Health care organizations and IT leaders should recognize that IT organizational attributes and cultures are created, intentionally or not, through the combined acts, speech, and behavior of its members. IT leaders mold culture every time they speak or don't speak, act or don't act, reward or punish, and hire or fail to hire.

IT organizations will struggle if they attempt to create a culture or character that is significantly different from that of the rest of the organization, particularly if members of IT have to interact with other members of the organization on any routine basis. The two different cultures are at risk of rejecting each other, often for reasons no more solid than "they are different."

Strategies regarding organizational attributes will identify and define important attributes and carry out the management initiatives deemed necessary to establish those attributes. These strategies should recognize that attributes change takes time and can be very difficult.

Observations on the Staff Component of the IT Asset. All elements of the IT asset are important. The failure or suboptimal condition of any element impairs the ability of IT to advance the organization. Each element needs strategic discussions and strategies directed toward improving it. Nonetheless, of all components of the assets, staff is the most important. Staff can create or alter all the other components, and the quality of the resulting creation depends heavily on the quality of the staff. The quality of the staff is not simply the quality of the IT talent (as good as it might be). The staff must be organized well, have "A-plus" competencies, and have all the desired attributes.

Governance

Governance refers to the principles, processes, and organization that govern the IT resources (Drazen and Staisor, 1995). Strategies regarding governance must address several issues:

- Who sets priorities for IT and how are those priorities set?
- Who is responsible for implementing information systems plans, and what principles will guide the implementation process?
- What organization structures are needed to support the linkage between IT and the rest of the organization?
- How are IT responsibilities distributed between IT and the rest of the organization and between central and "local" IT groups?
- How are IT budgets developed?
- What principles will govern the IT asset?

At its core, governance involves determining the distribution of the responsibility for making decisions, the scope of the decisions that can be made by different organizational functions, and the processes to be used for making decisions. Developing answers to the questions just listed can be a complex exercise.

Governance Characteristics. Well-developed governance mechanisms have several distinct characteristics:

• They are perceived as objective and fair. No governance mechanisms are free of politics, and some decisions will be made as part of "side deals." Nonetheless, governance should be viewed by organizational participants as fair, objective, appropriately public in its deliberations, and possessed of integrity. The ability of governance to govern is dependent on the willingness of organizational participants to be governed.

• They are efficient and timely. Governance mechanisms should arrive at decisions quickly, and the governance process should be efficient, eliminating as much bureaucracy as possible.

• They evolve appropriately. Governance will change as the organization and its environment changes. The advent of end-user computing, two decades ago, had an impact on IT governance leading to personal computer committees. Several organizations spun off portions of IT to support the organization's e-commerce undertakings. This spin-off is an effort, among other objectives, to "free" e-commerce initiatives from the normal "bureaucracy" of the organization's governance structures. The growing intertwining of information systems between partnering organizations will require new governance mechanisms to deal with interorganizational IT issues.

Linkage of Governance to Organizational Strategies. Governance should be heavily influenced by basic strategic objectives; for example, a desire to be integrated has ramifications for the design of governance. Some examples of governance derived from a strategic objective are presented in the sections that follow.

Governance to support the integration of an IDS might adopt the following objectives:

• Priorities should be developed by a central IDS IT committee to help ensure the perspective of overall integration, and initiatives that support integration should be given a higher priority than those that do not.
• IT budgets that are developed locally are subject to central approval.
• The IT plan must specify the means by which an integrated infrastructure and application suites will be achieved and the boundaries of that plan—for example, local organizations are free to select from a set of patient care system options, but whatever the selection, the patient care system must interface with the IDS clinical data repository.
• A centralized IT group must exist, and it has authority over local groups.
• Members of the IDS are constrained in their selection of applications to support ancillary departments to those that are on an "approved" list.
• Certain pieces of data, such as payer class or patient problems, and certain identifiers, such as patient identifier and provider identifier, have to use a common dictionary or standard.
• All IDS members must use a common e-mail system.

Governance to support the ability of the IDS member organizations to be locally responsive might select the following objectives:

- A small central IT group will be created to assist in local IT plan development; develop technical, data, and application standards; and perform technical research and development. This group will have an advisory and coordination relationship with the local IT organizations.
- Local IT steering committees will develop local IT plans according to processes and criteria defined locally. A central IT steering committee will review these plans, in an advisory role, to identify areas of potential redundancy or serious inconsistency.
- IT budgets are developed locally according to overall budget guidelines established centrally; examples are the rules for capitalizing new systems and the duration to use for depreciation.
- Certain pieces of data will be standardized as appropriate to ensure the ability of the IDS to prepare consolidated financial statements and patient activity counts.
- Local sites have the freedom, for example, to select any e-mail system, but that system must be able to send and receive messages using SMTP, and the e-mail system directory should be able to reveal itself to other e-mail directories.

Developing governance structures and approaches requires strategies that are driven by the need to achieve certain organizational objectives. Governance should not be developed purely for the purpose of performing some normative task; for example, all organizations have IT steering committees composed of a broad representation of senior leaders, and therefore so should we. An organizational objective of being locally responsive may mean that no central steering committee would exist or that its powers would be limited.

Several examples of governance strategies are discussed in the following sections.

Central and Local Responsibilities. Partners HealthCare undertook an examination of its IT governance structure in 1997. A critical question (typically faced by any organization with a corporate function and local business units) was, "What responsibilities should be given to corporate IT and what responsibilities should be given to the IT groups supporting local business units?"

The answer to this question must account for trade-offs between ensuring that business units have the flexibility to respond to local conditions and meet local operating targets and ensuring the overall ability to integrate the system and achieve systemwide efficiencies. The answer must recognize that the needs of community hospitals are different from those of academic medical centers. The answer must also understand that this is not purely a question of reporting relationships; the local IT groups report to the central IT group.

The following set of information systems operating principles was developed. The corporate IT function would have the following roles:

- Ensure functioning of a common core of applications and infrastructure
- Determine Partners-wide integration agenda
- Fund core operations function, IT-owned Partners-wide projects, and IT research and development
- Support and execute local integration initiatives
- Set minimum standards
- Deliver applications and new solutions
- Recommend Partners-wide IT capital budget
- Undertake research and development with a focused agenda of "breakthrough" high-value approaches and techniques

The business unit IT functions would have the following roles:

- Determine local "islands" of integration needs, priorities, pace, business case, and project funding
- Determine local applications needs, priorities, pace, business case, project funding, and implementation needs

In essence, the corporate function was very centralized. Business units would establish local plans and priorities (and fund them). The corporate function would execute those plans within the context of standards and an overall integration agenda.

IT Committee of the Board. Partners created a board-level committee on IT. (This committee is discussed in detail in the section on IT value later in this chapter.) The Partners board recognized the critical contribution of IT to Partners' strategies and ongoing operations. Realizing that the normal board agenda might not always allow sufficient time for discussion of important IT issues and that not all board members had extensive experience in IT, the board formed a committee of board members who were seasoned IT professionals (IT academics and CEOs from the IT industry). This committee would inform the board of its recommendations and assessments. The board improved its ability to govern IT by ensuring that thorough discussions of IT issues and strategies occurred at the trustee level.

IT Budget Development. In fiscal year 1999, Partners altered its approach to the development of the IT budget. (This alteration is also discussed in more detail in the section on IT value later in this chapter.) The change in the budget process led to users defending requests for new applications rather than IT. The change also eliminated the separate IT budget discussion and merged that discussion into the overall budget discussion. This change was designed to achieve several objectives. One was to shift the responsibility for defending and obtaining funds for new applications from IT to user management.

The Chief Information Officer

The role of the chief information officer (CIO), and the need for one, has been much discussed in the IT and management literature and at conferences over the past two decades. The CIO is regarded as the executive who would successfully lead the organization in its efforts to apply information technology to advance its strategies and can be viewed as a critical component of the IT asset.

In health care, surveys, such as those conducted by the College of Healthcare Information Management Executives (CHIME) (1998), have chronicled the evolution of the health care CIO. This evolution has included debates on CIO reporting relationships, salaries, titles, pedigrees (from outside health care or not), and the role of the CIO in organizational strategic planning.

A good CIO can be a significant asset to an organization. The CIO can

- Be a major contributor to organizational strategy development and apply business thinking and strategy formation skills that extend beyond his or her IT responsibilities
- Help the organization understand the potential of IT to make real and significant contributions to organizational plans, activities, and operations
- Be a leader, motivator, recruiter, and retainer of superior IT talent
- Ensure that the IT asset is robust, effective, efficient, and sustained
- Ensure that the IT organization runs effectively and efficiently

Earl and Feeny (1995) conducted a study of CIOs who "added value" to their respective organizations. They found that the value-adding CIOs

- Obsessively and continuously focus on business imperatives so that they focus the IT direction correctly
- Have delivery track records that cause IT performance problems to drop off of the management agenda
- Interpret, for the rest of the leadership, the meaning and nature of the IT success stories of other organizations
- Establish and maintain good working relationships with the members of the organization's leadership
- Establish and communicate the IT performance record

- Concentrate the IT development efforts on the areas of the organization where the most leverage is to be gained
- Work with the organization's leadership to develop a shared vision of the role and contribution of IT
- Make important general contributions to business thinking and operations

Earl and Feeny (1995) also found that the value-adding CIO, as a person, has integrity, is goal-directed, is experienced with IT, and is a good consultant and communicator. Organizations that have such a CIO tend to describe IT as critical to the organization, find that IT thinking is embedded in business thinking, note that IT initiatives are well focused, and speak highly of IT performance.

Organizational excellence in IT doesn't just happen. It is managed and led. If the organization decides that the effective application of IT is a major element of its strategies and plans, it will need a very good CIO. Failure to have such talent will severely hinder the organization's aspirations.

Although CIOs can be of great value, the health care CIO community, and some of its members, can hobble themselves and their potential for contributing to the organization by directing the conversation into areas of concern that do little to advance the organization. The health care CIO community often expresses specific concerns:

- Concerns about the reporting relationship of the CIO. Not everyone will report to the CEO (which is merciful to the CEO). The CIO needs access to the CEO but also needs a boss who is a good mentor, provides appropriate political support, and is genuinely interested in the application of IT. CFOs and COOs can be terrific in these regards.
- Concerns that the organization doesn't understand how hard the management and the implementation of the technology can be and how nefarious the vendor and consulting community can be. All members of the organization can drag out litanies that portray the general difficulty of life or the problems of changing large, unruly organizations or the failure of the rest of the world to appreciate the complexities and value of their profession. Part of the problem is that the organization, to a degree, doesn't care about the woes of a profession; it just wants the job to get done. And part of the problem is the CIO's failure to communicate well about the challenges posed by IT.
- Concerns about the lack of senior management interest in technologies and applications such as the clinical data repository, client-server technology, and object-oriented development environments. Management will care if it understands why it should care. Management is no more interested in CIO discussions of seemingly arcane and irrelevant aspects of the IT arena than it is in CFO

monologues on murky Medicare rulings or medical staff ramblings on the nuances of new clinical findings.

Asset Lessons Learned and Observations

In addition to the lessons and observations discussed so far in this chapter, two overall observations of the IT asset are necessary: the need for asset plans and caveats regarding asset investments.

Plans for the Asset

IT strategic plans invariably center on the applications that need to be implemented to further organizational goals. Though that focus is not inappropriate, these plans often give insufficient attention to describing the activities and resources needed to advance the nonapplication portion of the asset. (Moreover, the application portion of the plan is often an inventory of systems to be implemented with little analyses of fundamental characteristics of the application asset.)

On the one hand, one should not conclude that a solid infrastructure, terrific staff, well-crafted infrastructure, and high-quality data are a substitute for the need to deliver applications. On the other hand, it is difficult to deliver applications properly and consistently if the asset is in poor shape. In an analogous fashion, one may be able to force one's dreadfully out-of-shape body to hike twenty miles, but one might not be able to hike twenty miles day after day until the body's fitness is improved. Money invested in enhancing the asset can deliver more of a return than money invested in an application.

IT plans need to devote serious attention to the steps that will be taken, for example, to improve infrastructure agility, improve staff skills, enhance data quality, and streamline governance processes. These plans require serious strategic thinking. Ill-conceived analyses or half-baked strategies surrounding plans for IT governance or technical architecture, for example, can severely impede organization progress.

Asset Investment

A study by Strassmann (1990) examined the relationship between IT expenditures and organizational effectiveness. Data from *Information Week*'s survey of the top 100 best users of information technology was used to correlate IT expenditures per employee with profits per employee (see Figure 3.8). Strassman concluded that

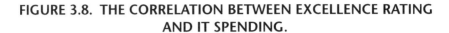

FIGURE 3.8. THE CORRELATION BETWEEN EXCELLENCE RATING AND IT SPENDING.

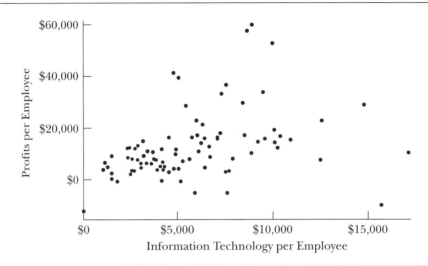

Source: P. Strassmann, *The Business Value of Computers* (New Canaan, Conn.: Information Economics Press, 1990), p. 52. Reprinted with permission.

there is no obvious direct relationship between expenditure and organizational performance. This finding has been corroborated in several other studies (see, for example, Keen, 1997).

This finding leads to several conclusions.

• Just because you spend more, there is no guarantee that the organization will be better off. There has never been a correlation between spending and outcomes. Paying more for care doesn't give one better care. Clearly, one can spend so little that nothing effective can be done. And one can spend so much that waste is guaranteed. But moving IT expenditures from 2 percent of the operating budget to 3 percent of the operating budget does not inherently lead to a 50 percent increase in desirable outcomes.

• Information technology is a tool, and its utility as a tool is largely determined by the tool users and their task. Spending a large amount of money on a chainsaw for someone who doesn't know how to use one is a waste. Spending more money for the casual saw user who trims an apple tree every now and then is also a waste. But a skilled logger might say that if the blade were longer and the engine more powerful, he would be able to cut 10 percent more trees in a given period of time. The investment needed to enhance the saw might lead to superior performance. Organizational effectiveness at applying IT has an enormous effect on the potential for a useful outcome from increased IT investment.

• Factors other than the appropriateness of the tool to the task influence the relationship between IT investment and organizational performance. Factors include the nature of the work—for example, IT is likely to have a greater impact on bank performance than on the performance of a consulting firm; the basis of competition in an industry—for example, cost per unit of manufactured output versus prowess of marketing; and an organization's relative competitive position in the market.

In health care, we often decry that while banks spend 8 to 10 percent of their revenue on IT, we spend only 2 to 3 percent. There are several reasons why that disparity exists (excluding the contention that physicians are technology Luddites):

• Health care has become competitive only recently.
• Health care organizations have only recently hit a scale where IT investments can have great leverage over organizational processes.
• The nature of information processing at a bank is less complex than health care and more amenable to today's IT solutions.

Regardless, there is no evidence that health care would be more effective and efficient if it spent four times as much on IT as it does now. Certainly, Strassmann's analysis wouldn't support the conclusion that more money leads to better performance.

IT-Centric Organizational Attributes

Several studies have examined organizations that have been particularly effective in the use of IT. Determining effectiveness is difficult, and the studies have defined it differently. Definitions have included organizations that have developed information systems that defined an industry, for example, the SABRE system; organizations that have the reputation of being effective over decades; and organizations that have had instances of exceptional IT innovation.

These studies have attempted to identify the factors or attributes of these organizations that have created the environment in which effectiveness occurred. In effect, the studies have sought to answer the question, "What organizational factors allow certain organizations to develop remarkable IT prowess?"

If an organization understands these attributes and desires to be very effective in its use of IT, it is in a position to develop strategies to create or modify its attributes. For example, one attribute is the strength of the working relationships between the IT function and the rest of the organization. If that relationship is weak or dysfunctional, strategies and plans can be implemented to improve the relationship.

We shall review four of these studies.

Financial Executives Research Foundation

The Financial Executives Research Foundation sponsored a study, conducted by Sambamurthy and Zmud (1996), on factors that led to the development of visionary IT applications. Visionary applications are

> applications that help managers make decisions, introduce new products and services more quickly and frequently, improve customer relations, and enhance the manufacturing process. Visionary IT applications seek to transform some of a firm's business processes in "framebreaking" ways. These applications create a variety of benefits to businesses that not only affect their current operations but also provide opportunities for new markets, strategies, and relationships [p. 1].

The study had findings in several areas.

Visionary Applications. Visionary applications focused on leveraging core business operations, enhancing decision making, improving customer service, and speeding up the ability to deliver new products and services. These applications were "platforms" that enabled the business to handle multiple work processes. An example of such a platform in health care is the computerized medical record.

The Justification Process. Visionary projects required the participation of four key players. Envisioners conceptualized the initial ideas for a project. Project champions were instrumental in selling the envisioners' ideas and value to senior executives. Executive sponsors provided champions with seed funding and political support. IT experts supplied the necessary technical vision and expertise to ensure that the idea would work.

Facilitating Investment in Visionary IT Applications. Several factors facilitate investment in visionary applications:

• A climate must exist that enables employees to have the power—and the support—to undertake visionary applications that often carry significant personal and organizational risk.

- Mechanisms need to exist to invest, continuously, in IT technical infrastructures.
- Coordinating mechanisms must be established to bring together envisioners, project champions, executive sponsors, and IT experts.
- The role of the CIO, in addition to that of an envisioner and IT expert, was to ensure that the envisioners' proposal furthered the interests of the business, to serve as architect and advocate for the corporate IT technical infrastructure, and to serve as the architect of IT-related coordinating mechanisms.

Rationale for Justifying Visionary IT Applications. Visionary IT applications were generally defended using two distinct strategies: their contribution to critical work processes or their support of a primary strategic driver. In addition to the discussion and analysis that would surround one of these two strategies, prototypes, best-practice visitations, and consultants would often be used to further organizational understanding of the proposed initiative.

Ross, Beath, and Goodhue

Ross, Beath, and Goodhue (1996) examined the factors that enable organizations to achieve long-term competitiveness in the application of IT. They identified the development and management of three key IT assets as critical to achieving a sustained IT-based competitive advantage.

Highly Competent IT Human Resources. A well developed IT human resource asset is one that "consistently solves business problems and addresses business opportunities through information technology" (p. 33). This asset has three dimensions:

- IT staff had the technical skills needed to craft and support applications and infrastructures and to understand and appropriately apply new technologies.
- IT staff had superior working relationships with the end-user community and were effective at furthering their own understanding of the business and its directions, cultures, work processes, and politics.
- IT staff were responsible—and knew that they were responsible—for solving business problems. This orientation goes beyond performing discreet tasks and leads IT staff to believe that they "own," and have the power to carry out, the challenge of solving business problems.

The Technology Asset. The technology asset consists of "sharable technical platforms and databases" (p. 33). The technology asset had two distinguishing characteristics:

- A well-developed technology architecture that defined the rules for the distribution of hardware, software, and support
- Standards that limit the technologies that will be supported

Failure to create a robust architecture can result in applications that are difficult to change, poorly integrated, expensive to manage, and unable to accommodate organizational growth (Weill and Broadbent, 1998). These limitations hinder the ability of the organization to advance. IT resources, efforts, and capital can be consumed by the difficulty of managing the current base of infrastructure and applications, and relatively modest advances can be too draining.

The Relationship Asset. When the relationship asset is strong, IT and the business unit management share the risk and responsibility for effective application of IT in the organization. A solid relationship asset is present when the business unit is accountable for all IT projects and top management leads the IT priority-setting process.

The study noted the interrelationships between the assets. IT and user relationships are strengthened by the presence of a strong IT staff. A well-developed, agile infrastructure enables the IT staff to execute project delivery at high levels and be more effective at solving business problems.

McKenney, Copeland, and Mason

McKenney, Copeland, and Mason (1995) studied the factors that allowed managerial teams to create and implement innovative information systems. They were particularly interested in examples where the resulting information systems became the dominant design in a particular industry. They studied American Airlines, Bank of America, the United States Automobile Association, Baxter Travenol/American Hospital Association, and Frito-Lay.

Their study came to interesting conclusions in several areas.

Management Team. All IT innovations were led proactively by a management team driven to change its processes through the means of information technology. The management team had to encompass three essential roles:

- The CEO or other senior executive who was both visionary and a good businessperson. This person had sufficient power and prestige to drive technological innovation.
- The "technology maestro," often the CIO, who had a remarkable combination of business acumen and technological competency. The CIO must deliver the system and recruit, energize, and lead a superb technical team.

- The technical team who understood how to apply the technology in innovative ways and was capable of developing new business processes that leverage the technology.

In addition to exceptional competency in each role, there was a rare chemistry between the players in the roles. A change in a role's incumbent often stalled the innovation. This suggests that a great CIO in one setting may not be a great CIO in another setting.

Evolution of the Innovation. The innovative systems evolved over time and generally went through several phases:

1. A business crisis develops, such as Bank of America's being overwhelmed by the volume of paper transactions, and a search begins for an IT solution.
2. IT competency is built as research is conducted in search of potential IT solutions, particularly the application of new technology.
3. The IT solution is planned and developed.
4. IT is used to restructure the organization and processes and to lead changes in organizational strategies.
5. The strategy evolves, and the systems are refined. Competitors begin to emulate the success.

In these phases, the capabilities of the technology heavily influenced and constrained the operational changes that were envisioned and implemented.

This series of phases occurs over the course of five to seven years, reflecting the magnitude of the organizational change and the time required to experiment with, understand, and implement new information technology. This interval suggests that CIO (or CEO) average tenures of three years or less risk thwarting the organization's ability to make truly innovative IT-based transformations.

Capitalizing on IT Innovation. A particular IT innovation was identified by the organization, early in the life of the technology, as being the breakthrough necessary to resolve the business crisis or challenge. In the cases studied, the breakthrough was the transistor, time-sharing, and cheap mass storage. Today the technology might be the Internet or voice recognition.

Weill and Broadbent

Weill and Broadbent (1998) studied firms that "consistently achieve more business value for their information technology investment" (p. 65). Their study noted that these organizations were excellent or above average in five characteristics.

Greater Top Management Commitment to Information Technology. The leadership of the organization was committed to the strategic and effective application of IT. This commitment was widely known within the organization. Management participated actively in IT strategy discussions, thoughtfully assessed the business contribution of proposed IT investments, and provided seed funding to innovative and experimental IT projects.

Less Political Turbulence. IT investments often serve to integrate processes and groups throughout the organization. Political conflict reduces the likelihood and success of interdisciplinary initiatives. IT investments can require that the proposals of one part of the organization be funded at the expense of other parts or other proposed non-IT initiatives. Political turbulence can reduce the likelihood that such "disproportionate" investments will occur.

More Satisfied Users. If the organization's staff have had good experiences with IT projects, they are more likely to view IT as something that can help their endeavors rather than a burden or an anchor.

Integrated Business Information Technology Planning. Organizations that do a very good job at aligning the IT plans and strategies with the overall organizational plans and strategies will be more effective with IT than those that do not align well.

More Experience. Organizations that are experienced in their use and application of the technology, and have had success in those experiences will be more thoughtful and focused in their continued application of IT. They will have a better understanding of the technology's capabilities and limitations. Users and their IT colleagues will have a better understanding of their respective needs and roles and the most effective ways of working together on initiatives.

Summary of Studies

The four studies just discussed suggest that organizations that aspire to effectiveness and innovation in their application of IT must take steps to ensure that the core capacity of the organization, for IT effectiveness, is developed such that high levels and sustained progress can be achieved. The development of this capacity is a different challenge than identifying specific opportunities to use IT in the course of improving core processes or ensuring that the IT agenda is aligned with the organizational agenda. As an analogy, a runner's training, injury management, and diet are designed to ensure the core capacity to run a marathon. This capacity development is different from the discussion of the strategy of running a specific marathon, which must consider the nature of the course, the competing runners, and the weather.

Though reaching somewhat different conclusions (resulting to a degree from different study questions), the four studies reached consensus in several areas:

• Individuals and leadership matter. It is critical that the organization possess talented, skilled, and experienced individuals. These individuals will occupy a variety of roles: CEO, CIO, IT staff, user middle management. These individuals must be strong contributors. Though such an observation may seem trite, too often organizations, dazzled by the technology or the glorified experiences of others, embark on technology crusades and substantive investments for which they have insufficient talent or leadership to effect well.

Leadership, in these studies, was essential. This leadership is needed on the part of organizational senior management (or executive sponsors), the CIO, and the project team. This leadership understood the vision, communicated the vision, was able to recruit and motivate a team, and had the staying power to see the innovation through several years of work and disappointments, setbacks, and political problems along the way.

• Relationships are crucial. In addition to strong individual players, the team must be strong. There are critical senior executive, IT executive, and project team roles that must be filled by highly competent individuals, and great chemistry must exist between the individuals in the distinct roles. Substituting team members, even involving a replacement by an equally strong individual, can diminish the team. This is true in IT innovation just as it is true in sports. Political turbulence diminished the ability to develop a healthy set of relationships among organizational players.

• The technological and technical infrastructure both enables and hinders. New technologies can provide new opportunities for organizations to embark on major transformations of their activities. This implies that while CIOs must have superior business and clinical understandings, they must also have a superior understanding of the technology. This should not imply that they can rewrite operating systems as well as the best system programmers, but it does mean that they must have an excellent understanding of the maturity, capabilities, and possible evolutions of information technology. Several innovations occurred because the IT group was able to identify and adopt an emerging technology that could make a significant contribution to addressing a current organizational challenge.

The studies stress the importance of well-developed technical architecture. Great architecture matters. Possessing state-of-the-art technology can be far less important than a well-architected infrastructure.

• The organization must encourage innovation. The organization's (and the IT organization's) culture and leadership must encourage creativity and experimentation. This encouragement needs to be practical and goal-directed; there must be a real business problem, crisis, or opportunity, and the project needs budgets, political protection, and deliverables.

• True innovation takes time. Creating visionary applications or industry-dominant designs or an exceptional IT asset takes time and a lot of work. The organizations studied by McKenney, Copeland, and Mason often took five to seven years for the innovation to fully mature and the organization to recast itself. The applications and designs will proceed through phases that are as normative as the passage from infancy to adulthood. Innovation, like the maturation of a human being, will see some variation in the timing, depth, and success at moving through phases.

• Evaluation of IT opportunities must be thoughtful. The visionary and dominant design IT innovations studied were analyzed and studied thoroughly. Nonetheless, the organizations engaged in these innovations understood that a large element of vision, management instinct, and "feel" guided the decision to initiate investment and continue investment. An organization that has had more experience with IT and more successful experiences will be more effective in the evaluation (and execution) of IT initiatives.

• Processes, data, and differentiation formed the basis of the innovation. All of these examples were based on a fundamental understanding of current organizational limitations. Innovations were directed to focus on those core elements, identified in Chapter Two as the basis for achieving an IT-based advantage: significant leveraging of processes, expanding and capitalizing on the ability to gather critical data, and achieving a high level of organizational differentiation. Often an organization pursued all three simultaneously. At times the organization evolved from one basis to another as the competition responded or as it recognized new leverage points.

• Alignment was mature and strong. The alignment of the IT activities and the business challenges or opportunities was strong. It was also mature in the sense that this alignment depended on close working relationships rather than methodologies.

• The IT asset was critical. Strong IT staff, well-designed IT governance, well-crafted architecture, and a superb CIO were critical attributes. There is substantial overlap between the factors identified in these studies and the components of the IT asset.

The Question of Value

To this point, we have discussed the alignment of IT with the strategies of the organization and the need to develop strategies for the IT asset and IT-centric organizational capabilities. Strategy and execution failures in any of these areas can diminish the value or return that an organization receives from its IT investments. Next, we explore the question of value in more detail, focusing on factors that can reduce the likelihood of "value realization." The discussion will elaborate on some of the factors already discussed and examine additional "value dilution" factors.

The leaders of health care organizations often face the challenge of realizing value from their IT investments. The leaders may make a series of observations.

- The magnitude of the IT operating and capital budgets is large. IT operations may consume 2 to 3 percent of the total operating budget, and IT may claim 15 to 30 percent of all capital. Although 2 to 3 percent may seem small, it can make the difference between a negative operating margin and a positive margin. Insurance companies may spend 50 to 80 percent of capital on IT, but a 15 to 30 percent IT expenditure for providers invariably means that funding for biomedical equipment (which can mean new revenue) and buildings (which improve the patient- and staff-friendliness of the organization and support the growth of clinical services) are diminished.

- The projected growth in IT budgets exceeds the growth in other budget categories. Provider organizations may permit overall operating budgets to increase at a rate close to the inflation rate (currently 3 to 4 percent). However, expenditures on IT often experience growth rates of 12 to 15 percent. At some point, an organization will note that the IT budget growth rate may singlehandedly lead to insolvency.

- Regardless of the amount spent, the leaders feel that not enough is being spent. Worthwhile proposals go unfunded every year. Infrastructure replacement and upgrades seems never-ending; "I thought we upgraded our network two years ago. Are you back already?"

- It is difficult to evaluate IT capital requests. At times this difficulty is a reflection of a poorly written or fatuous proposal. However, it can be difficult to compare a proposal that is directed to improve service with one directed to improve care quality or one directed to increase revenue or one necessary to achieve some level of regulatory compliance.

- The leaders, asked to list three instances over the past five years where IT investments have resulted in clear and unarguable returns to the organization, may return blank stares. However, the conversation may be difficult to stop when they are asked to list three major IT investment disappointments that have occurred over the past five years.

Why does this happen? And what can be done to improve the return on the IT investment?

Real Value

There are four types of IT value that can be realized by organizations:

- Tangible, measurable improvements in organizational performance have occurred—for example, reductions in medical errors, reductions in costs, improvements in service, and increases in revenue.
- The organization has been "transformed" to acquire critical attributes—for example, IT has been a critical component of an organization's efforts to become more service-oriented or agile or to move toward protocol-driven care.
- The organization has learned how to be more effective in applying IT; in other words, IT application has become an organizational competency.
- IT functions effectively and efficiently.

The first two types of value are generally viewed in the context of IT-strategy alignment; the latter two factors have been the focus of this chapter.

If we home in on the first category, which is generally where organizational leaders will focus, there is clear evidence that IT investments can provide value.

Figure 3.9 provides a Partners analysis of actual costs, comparing the manual cost to determine patient eligibility for coverage to the cost to perform the same task using two different approaches to an insurance electronic data interchange. In one of the approaches (the one used by Partners), there is a large up-

FIGURE 3.9. THREE APPROACHES TO ELIGIBILITY TRANSACTION COSTS.

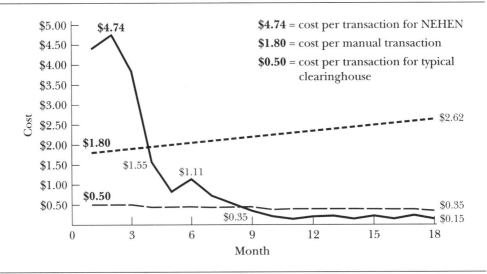

front capital investment, while in the other approach, there is an ongoing per transaction fee. The analysis shows that the cost can be reduced from $2.62 per transaction to 35 cents per transaction for one approach and 15 cents per transaction for the other approach. Both approaches achieve a significant decrease in the cost of supporting the transaction.

Figure 3.10 depicts a Partners analysis of the costs and dollar benefits of the computerized patient record (CPR). This analysis is based on the experiences of Partners' physician's use of a record. The cost of the record, amortized over five years, varies from $4,000 per physician FTE per year to $6,000 per physician FTE per year. The difference in cost reflects variations in workstation density and the level of implementation support. The dollar benefits range from $9,000 to $19,000 per physician FTE per year. These benefits can be achieved through reduction in transcription costs and record retrieval costs, improved conformance to ordering from approved formularies in cases where risk is shared, and improved billing accuracy.

Figure 3.11 depicts a 55 percent reduction in serious medication errors that resulted from the implementation of inpatient provider order entry at the Brigham and Women's Hospital (Bates and others, 1998). The order entry system highlighted, at the time of ordering, possible drug allergies, drug interactions, and drug-lab result problems.

Figure 3.12 depicts the impact of providing knowledge resources through an extranet for Partners community physicians who are members of Partners Community HealthCare, Inc. (PCHI), the subsidiary of Partners that manages its network of community physicians. Prior to the introduction of PCHInet, and six months after its implementation, the physician-users were asked to define their

FIGURE 3.10. COST-BENEFIT ANALYSIS OF THE COMPUTERIZED PATIENT RECORD.

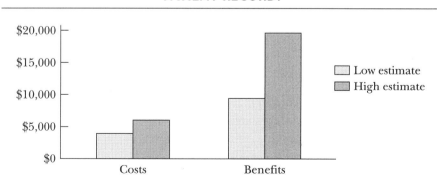

FIGURE 3.11. SERIOUS MEDICATION ERROR REDUCTION.

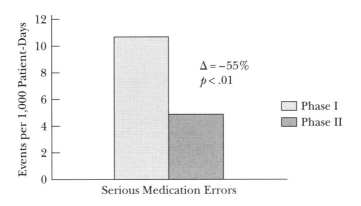

Source: Data from D. W. Bates and others, "Effect of Computerized Physician Order Entry and a Team Intervention on Prevention of Serious Medication Errors." *Journal of the American Medical Association,* 1998, *280,* 1311–1316. Used with permission.

FIGURE 3.12. PCHINET KNOWLEDGE RESOURCES.

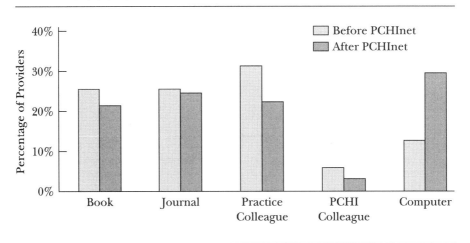

major sources of information when confronted with a question about the treatment of their patients. The computer as a source increased from 11 percent to 29 percent. This usage increase enables Partners to direct physicians to a set of information that is viewed, by the medical leadership, as being the most authoritative.

Finally, the impact of radiology Picture Archival and Communication System (PACS) implementation, measured one year after going filmless at the Massachusetts General Hospital (MGH), is presented in Table 3.2. The impact is diverse: cost reductions, service improvements, and productivity gains.

These data, and others like them seen at other organizations, enable one to draw several conclusions:

- The value from IT investments can be real and at times dramatic.
- The value across investments is diverse, making it difficult to compare investments.
- The value of any one investment, for example, PACS, can be diverse, making it difficult to distill the investment to a single number or single kind of analysis, such as return-on-investment analysis.

Why Does the IT Investment Fail to Deliver Returns?

If the value can be real, why does one hear management voicing so many concerns? There are several reasons that IT investments become simply IT expenses:

- We don't establish a clear linkage between IT investments and organizational strategy.
- We ask the wrong question.
- We often conduct the wrong analyses.
- We often don't state our goals.
- We don't manage the outcomes.
- We leap to inappropriate solutions.
- We mangle management of the project.
- We haven't learned from studies of IT effectiveness.

Let us examine each reason in turn.

TABLE 3.2. THE IMPACT OF PACS.

Total reduction in MGH radiology operating cost	$1.5 million per year
Average decrease in report turnaround time at Chelsea Health Center	74 hours to 4 hours
Average time saved for "image-intense" specialists such as neurosurgeons	2 hours per day

We Don't Establish a Clear Linkage Between Investments and Strategy. The linkage between the IT investments and the organizational strategy was discussed in Chapter Two. As noted in this chapter, there can be strategy formulation and implementation failures in both the overall organizational strategy and the related IT strategy. Even if the IT organization is executing well, it may be working on the wrong things or trying to support a flawed overall organizational strategy.

Linkage failures can occur for a variety of reasons, including the following:

- The organizational strategy is no more than a slogan or a buzzword, having the depth of a bumper sticker, making any investment toward it ill-advised.
- The IT department thinks it understands the strategy but doesn't, resulting in an implementation of an IT version of the strategy rather than the organization's version.
- The strategists won't engage in the IT discussion, forcing the IT leaders into the role of mind readers.
- The linkage is superficial—for example, "Patient care systems can reduce nursing labor costs, but we haven't thought through how that will happen."
- The IT strategy conversation is separated from the normal strategy conversation, as through the creation of an information systems steering committee, reducing the likelihood of alignment.
- The organizational strategy evolves faster than IT can respond.

We Ask the Wrong Question. The question "What is the ROI of a computer system?" should be asked only rarely. It makes about as much sense as the question "What is the ROI of a chain saw?" If one wants to make a dress, a chain saw is a waste of money. If one wants to cut down some trees, one can begin to think about the return on a chain saw investment and compare that investment to one in an ax. If the chain saw were to be used by one's ten-year-old child, the investment might be ill-advised. If the chain saw were to be used by a skilled lumberjack, the investment might be worthwhile.

One can only determine the ROI of an investment in a tool if one knows the task to be performed and the skill level of the participants who are to perform it. Moreover, a positive ROI is not an inherent property of an IT investment. Once implemented, no computer genie arrives, waves a magic wand, and miraculously ROI occurs. One has to manage a return into existence.

Hence instead of asking, "What is the ROI of a computer system?" one should ask a series of questions such as these:

- What are the steps to take and the investments, including IT, to make in order to achieve our goals?

- Which manager is responsible for the achievement of these goals? Does this manager have our confidence?
- Do the cost, risk, and time frame for the implementation of the set of investments, including the IT investment, seem appropriate in light of our goals?
- Have we assessed the trade-offs and opportunity costs?
- Are we comfortable with our ability to execute?

We Often Conduct the Wrong Analyses. There are times when ROI is the appropriate investment analysis technique. If a set of investments, including the IT component, is intended to reduce clerical staff, ROI can be calculated. However, there are times when the ROI is clearly inappropriate. What is the ROI of e-mail or word processing? One could calculate the ROI, but it is hard to imagine an organization basing its investment decision on that analysis. Would a ROI analysis have captured the strategic value of the American Airlines SABRE system or the value of automated teller machines? Few strategic IT investments have impacts that are fully captured by a ROI. Moreover, the strategic impact is rarely fully understood until years later. Whatever ROI analysis might have been done would have invariably been wrong.

The techniques used to assess IT investments should vary by the type of initiatives or objectives that the IT investment intends to support. One technique does not fit all IT investments. According to Quinn and others (1994), there are six categories of IT investments.

Infrastructure. IT investments can be infrastructure that enables other investments or applications to be implemented and deliver desired capabilities. Examples of infrastructure include data communication networks, personal computers, and clinical data repositories. A delivery-system-wide network enables one to implement applications to consolidate clinical laboratories, establish organizationwide e-mail, and share patient health data between providers.

It is difficult to assess the impact or value of infrastructure investments quantitatively, for the following reasons:

- They enable other applications. Without those applications, infrastructure has no value. Hence infrastructure value is indirect and depends on application value.
- The ability to allocate infrastructure value across applications is difficult. Of the millions of dollars invested in a data communication network, how much of that investment can be allocated to the ability to create delivery-system-wide electronic medical records may be difficult or impossible to determine.
- As was discussed earlier in this chapter, a good IT infrastructure is often determined by its agility, potency, and ability to facilitate integration of applications.

It is very difficult to assign return-on-investment numbers or any meaningful "value" number to some of these characteristics. What is the value of being able to speed up the time it takes to develop and enhance applications thanks to agility?

Information system infrastructure is as hard to evaluate as other organizational infrastructure, such as having talented, educated staff. As with other infrastructure:

- Evaluation is often instinctive and experientially based.
- In general, underinvesting can severely limit the organization.
- Investment decisions are made between alternatives that are assessed on the basis of their ability to achieve agreed-on goals. These goals may be difficult to quantify in terms of dollars. Examples include moving images across the system, high availability of information systems, and rapid application development.

Mandated. Information system investment may be necessary because of mandated initiatives. Examples of mandated initiatives may include reporting of quality data to accrediting organizations, required changes in billing formats, or compliance with the Health Insurance Portability and Accountability Act (HIPAA).

Assessing these initiatives is generally approached by identifying the alternative that costs the least and is the quickest to implement while achieving some level of compliance.

Cost Reduction. Information system investments directed to cost reduction are generally highly amenable to return-on-investment and other quantifiable impact analyses. The ability to conduct a quantifiable ROI analysis is rarely the question. The ability of management to effect the predicted cost reduction or avoidance is often a far more germane question.

Specific New Products and Services. IT can be critical to the development of new products and services. At times the information system delivers the new service or is itself the product. Examples of information-system-based new services include bank cash management programs and credit card–airline mileage linkage programs. In health care, a new service may be Web access, by patients, to guidelines and consumer-oriented medical texts.

For some of these new products and services, one can quantifiably assess these opportunities in terms of return. These assessments include analyses of potential revenues, either directly from the service or service-induced utilization of other products and services. A return-on-investment analysis will need to be supplemented by techniques such as sensitivity analyses of consumer responses.

Despite the analyses, the value of the investment usually has a speculative component. This component includes consumer utilization, competitor response, and impact on related businesses.

Quality Improvement. Information system investments are often directed to improving the quality of service or medical care. These investments may intend to reduce waiting times, improve physicians' ability to locate information, improve treatment outcomes, or reduce errors in treatment.

Evaluation of these initiatives, though quantifiable, is generally done in terms of service parameters that are known or believed to be important determinants of organizational success. As was discussed in Chapter Two, these parameters can be measures of aspects of organizational processes that customers encounter and are used by them to judge the organization, such as waiting times in the physician's office.

A quantifiable dollar outcome of service or care quality improvement can be very difficult to achieve. Service quality is often necessary to protect current business, and the effect of a failure to continuously improve service or medical care can be difficult to project.

Major Strategic Initiative. Strategic initiatives in IT are intended to significantly change the competitive position of the organization or redefine the core nature of the enterprise. In health care, information systems are rarely the centerpiece of organizational redefinition. However, other industries have attempted IT-centric transformations. Amazon.com mounted an effort to transform retailing. Schwab.com was an undertaking intended to redefine the brokerage industry through the use of the World Wide Web.

There can be an ROI core or component to these analyses in that they often involve major reshaping or reengineering of fundamental organizational processes. However, assessing the ROI of these initiatives and related information systems with any sort of accuracy can be very difficult. Several factors contribute to this difficulty:

- The initiatives usually recast the company's markets and its roles. The outcome of the recasting, albeit visionary, can be difficult to see with clarity and certainty.
- The recasting is evolutionary; the organization learns and alters itself as it progresses over what are often lengthy periods of time. It is difficult to be prescriptive about this evolutionary process. Most integrated delivery systems are confronting this phenomenon.
- Market and competitor responses can be difficult to predict.

We Often Don't State Our Goals. IT proposals are often accompanied by statements about the positive contributions that the investment will make to organizational performance. But the proposals are not always accompanied by specific numerical goals for this improvement. If we intend to reduce medical errors, will we reduce errors by 50 percent or 80 percent or some other number? If we intend to reduce claims denials, will we reduce them to 5 percent or 2 percent? And how much revenue will be realized as a result of these denials?

Failure to be numerically explicit about goals can create three fundamental value problems:

- We may not know how well we perform now. If we don't know our current error rate or denial rate, it is hard to believe that we have studied the problem well enough to be fairly sure that an IT investment will help achieve the desired gains. The IT proposal sounds more like a guess of what is needed.
- We may never know whether we got the desired value or not. If we don't state a goal, we'll never know whether the 20 percent reduction in errors is as far as we can go or whether we are halfway to our desired goal. We don't know whether we should continue to work on the error problem or whether we should move on to the next performance issue.
- It will be difficult to hold people accountable for performance improvement if we are unable to track how well they are doing.

We Don't Manage the Outcomes. Related to the problem with goals, we often don't manage the outcome into existence. Once the project is approved and the system is up, management goes off to the next challenge seemingly unaware that the real work of value realization has just begun.

Figure 3.13 depicts the reduction in days in accounts receivable (AR) at a Partners physician practice. During the interval of time depicted, a new practice management system was implemented. One doesn't see a precipitous decline in days in AR in the time immediately following the implementation. One does see a progressive improvement in days in AR because someone was managing that improvement.

We Leap to Inappropriate Solutions. At times the IT discussion of a new application succumbs to advanced states of technical arousal. Project participants become overwhelmed by the prospect of using sexy new technology and state-of-the-art gizmos and lose their senses and understanding of why they are having the discussion in the first place. Sexiness and state-of-the-art-ness become the criteria for making system decisions.

FIGURE 3.13. REDUCING DAYS IN ACCOUNTS RECEIVABLE.

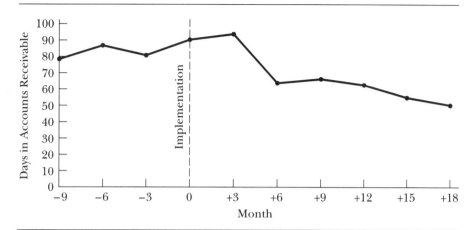

In addition, the comparison of two alternative vendor products can get lost in the features beauty contest. One product outdazzles another. The discussion devolves into a features war.

Both sexiness and features have their place in the system selection decision. However, they are secondary to the discussion that centers on the capabilities needed to effect specific performance goals. Sexiness and features can be irrelevant to the performance improvement discussion.

We Mangle Management of the Project. One guaranteed way to reduce value is to mangle the management of the implementation project. Implementation failures or significant budget and timetable overruns or really unhappy users all dilute value.

Projects become mangled for many reasons, including these:

- Project scope is poorly defined.
- Accountability is unclear.
- Project participants are marginally skilled.
- The magnitude of the task is underestimated.
- Users feel like victims rather than participants.
- All the world has a vote and can vote at any time.

We Haven't Learned from Studies of IT Effectiveness. Organizations fail to invest in IT capabilities as discussed earlier in this chapter. As a result, they increase the likelihood that the percentage of projects that fail to deliver value will be higher than it should be.

Studies on IT Value Achievement

A study by Quinn and others (1994) found that the major contributors to failure to achieve a solid return on IT investments were the following factors:

- A suboptimal organizational strategy or organizational assessment of the competitive environment. Insufficient return occurs because the overall strategy is wrong.
- An acceptable strategy with inappropriately defined associated IT capabilities. The information system, if it is solving a problem, is solving the wrong problem.
- Failure to identify and draw together all investments and initiatives necessary to carry out the organization's plans. The IT investment falters because other changes, such as reorganization or reengineering, fail to occur.
- Failure to execute the plan well. Poor planning or less than stellar management can diminish the return from any investment.

Value can be diluted by factors beyond the organization's control. Weill and Broadbent (1998) noted that the more strategic the IT investment, the more its value can be diluted. An IT investment directed to increasing market share can have its value diluted by non-IT decisions and events, including pricing decisions, the actions of competitors, and the reactions of customers. IT investments that are less strategic but have business value, such as improving nursing productivity, can also be diluted by factors outside the control of management, for example, shortages of nursing staff. The value of an IT investment directed toward improving the characteristics of the infrastructure can be diluted by factors unrelated to the IT organization, such as unanticipated technology immaturity or business difficulties encountered by a vendor.

The IT investment value challenge plagues all industries. This is not a problem peculiar to health care. The challenge has been with us for forty years, ever since organizations began to spend money on big mainframes. This challenge is complex and persistent, and we shouldn't believe that we can solve it. We should believe that we can do better at dealing with it.

Health care organization leadership often feels ill equipped to address the IT investment value challenge. However, no new management techniques are required to evaluate IT plans, proposals, and progress. Leaders are often asked to make decisions that involve strategic hunches (a strategy to develop a continuum of care) where they may have limited domain knowledge (new surgical modalities) and where the value is fuzzy (improved morale). Organizational leaders should treat IT investments no differently from these other types of investments; if they don't understand, believe, or trust the proposal or proponent, they shouldn't approve it.

And if they don't understand the CIO, it is the CIO's fault and not the fault of other members of the leadership team.

Additional Steps to Increase Value Delivery

There are several steps that organizations can take to improve the realization of value from their IT investments. Chapter Two and this chapter discussed the need for alignment and IT asset investment in order to enhance value realization. Chapter Four provides examples of strategic thinking surrounding several types of IT investments being made at Partners.

Some additional steps that can be taken by organizational leaders to enhance value realization are discussed next.

Hone Listening Skills. Critical listening skills can be applied to IT presentations and discussions. When listening to discussions of the IT strategic plan, ask:

- Is it clear how the plan advances the organization's strategy?
- Is it clear how (and to what degree) care will improve, costs will be reduced, or service will be improved?
- Are senior leaders, whose business areas are the focus of the IT plan, clearly supportive and capable of giving the presentation themselves?

As leaders listen to the presentation of a specific IT project proposal, they should ask all the questions we just examined:

- Are we asking the right question?
- Have we conducted the appropriate analyses?
- Have we stated our goals?

and so on through the list.

Create an IT Subcommittee of the Board. The creation of an IT subcommittee of the board can enhance organizational efforts to achieve value from IT investments. At times the leaders of organizations are uncomfortable with some or all of the IT conversation. They may not understand why infrastructure is so expensive or why large implementations can take so long and cost so much. The creation of a subcommittee that has members more experienced with these discussions can help ensure that hard questions are being asked and that the answers are sound.

The leaders should not believe that such a subcommittee gets them off the hook for having to deal with IT issues. Rather the committee should be viewed as a way for the leaders to continue their efforts to become more knowledgeable and comfortable with the IT conversation.

A charter for such a committee could be as follows:

- Review and critique IT application, technical, and organizational strategies.
- Review and critique overall IT tactical plans and budgets.
- Discuss and provide advice on major IT issues and challenges.
- Explore opportunities to leverage industry partnerships.

Committee members can be a combination of trustees, invited external participants, IT leaders, and organizational leaders.

Committee agenda items could include the following:

- Internet strategy
- Obtaining value from clinical information systems
- Financial system long-term plans
- IT staff recruitment and retention issues
- Annual IT budget

Revamp IT Budget Development. The approach an organization uses to develop its IT budget can assist in achieving value. The approach described here was adopted by Partners for the fiscal 1999 budget process and has been reasonably successful.

Information Systems submits an operating budget to support the applications and infrastructure that will be in place as of the beginning of the fiscal year. This budget is targeted to be an 8 percent increase over the support budget for the prior fiscal year. The 8 percent increase reflects inflation, merit programs, a recognition that new systems were implemented during the fiscal year and will require support, and an acknowledgment that infrastructure (workstations, remote locations and storage) consumption will increase by an average of 10 percent. Within the 8 percent, IT is also expected to have plans to carry out a 2 percent reduction in operating expenses.

Capital to support applications and infrastructure that will be in place as of the beginning of the fiscal year should be the same as what was budgeted in the prior fiscal year.

The submitted IT budget proposes no new initiatives for the fiscal year.

If there is organizational interest in new applications, such as contract management or laboratory systems, or infrastructure, such as improved security and new storage technologies, these requests must go through the following steps:

- The project must be sponsored, presented, and defended by a non-IT person except for infrastructure, which the CIO must present.
- The presentation of these projects must occur as part of the overall organizational capital and operating budget development process and meetings; there is no separate track for IT discussions. In other words, budget requests for new IT applications are reviewed in the same conversation that discusses budget requests for new clinical services.
- The level of analytical rigor required by the IT projects is the same as required of any other requested budget item.
- If the IT project is approved, the budget is added to the IT support budget.

This process requires that a sponsor, for example, a clinical vice president, defend his or her specific IT request in front of colleagues. The sponsor will determine whether to present the IT proposal or some other, perhaps non-IT, proposal. The sponsor will decide if the IT investment should be made instead of other investment requests that they are being asked to defend.

Both sponsor and colleagues know that if the IT proposal is approved, there will be less money available for other initiatives. The defender also knows that the value being promised must be delivered, or his or her credibility next year will be diminished. The defender also learns how to be comfortable presenting IT proposals.

Fundamentally, this process gets IT out of the role of defending other people's improvement initiatives. IT must still support the budget requests of others by providing data on the costs and capabilities of the proposed applications and the time frames and resources required to implement them. If IT believes that the proposed initiative lacks merit or is too risky, it needs to ensure that its opinions are heard during the budget approval process.

This process also means that IT requests are treated no differently from other budget requests.

IT faces the risk that the budget defense process yields no new IT initiatives for the next fiscal year. Distressing though this prospect may be to IT, it may be a very reasonable organizational conclusion.

Other Value Suggestions. IT should develop a communication plan. This plan should, for the year ahead, indicate which presentations will be made in which forums and how often IT-centric columns will appear in organizational newsletters. The plan should list three or so major themes that will be the focus of the communication plan—for example, Internet strategies or efforts to improve IT service. Communication plans recognize that value may be being delivered but that the organization is not fully aware of it.

The IT organization should benchmark, comparing itself to other organizations. Benchmarking can be in the form of participation in industry surveys or commissioned studies. Benchmarking can at times be painful, as weaknesses are highlighted. But self-criticism and continuous efforts to improve performance are crucial contributors to ongoing value delivery.

Postimplementation audits should be conducted of a sample of new system implementations. These audits seek to understand if the project goals have been achieved and, if they have not, what steps need to be taken to achieve them.

Business value should be celebrated. Organizations usually hold parties shortly after applications "go live." These parties are appropriate; a lot of people worked very hard to get the system up and running and used. However, up and running and used does not mean that value has been delivered. In addition to go-live parties, organizations should consider business value parties, celebrations conducted once the value has been achieved. Go-live parties as the end point send the signal that implementation is the end point of the IT initiative.

When possible, projects should have short deliverable cycles. In other words, rather than waiting twelve months or eighteen months for the organization to see the first fruits of its application system labors, efforts should be made to deliver a sequence of smaller implementations every quarter. Rather than a big-bang delivery of 100 percent of features, strive for four 25 percent minibangs. The shortened cycles, which are not always doable, enable the organization to achieve some value earlier rather than later, support organizational learning about what system capabilities are really important versus those that were thought to be important, and create the appearance (not to be underestimated) of more value delivery.

Assessment of the IT Function

A wide range of analysis and academic study has been directed to the broad question "How do we assess the value of our overall investments in IT?" This question is generally directed at assessing the value of the aggregate IT investment or the contribution of the IT organization. This is different from assessing the value of an initiative or a specific investment and at times more complex.

Developing a definitive, accurate, and well-accepted way to assess IT value has eluded the industry and may continue to be elusive. Nonetheless, there are some basic questions that can be asked. Interpreting the answers is a subjective exercise, making it difficult to derive numerical scores. Bresnahan (1998) suggests five questions:

- How does IT influence the customer experience? Do patients and physicians, for example, find that organizational processes are more efficient, less error-prone, and more convenient?

- Does IT enable or retard growth? Can the IT organization support effectively the demands of a merger? Can IT support the creation of clinical product lines, for example, Cardiology, across the IDS?
- Does IT favorably affect productivity?
- Does IT advance organizational innovation and learning?
- How well is IT run?

The following is a crude but effective way of assessing the IT function (Glaser, 1991):

- Ask three members of the management team to identify the major IT initiatives for the next year. Inconsistent answers or blank stares indicate a failure in the IT planning process.
- Review the expectations that were set for the last two systems you purchased. Ask for an assessment of the extent to which the goals were met and whether the implementation was on time and on budget.
- Ask for information to support two upcoming decisions. See whether, how quickly, and at what costs the requests can be satisfied.
- Ask your CIO for his or her assessment of the role of Internet in the organization. Did you understand the answer? Does the response seem thoughtful?
- Ask the CIO how your level of IT expenditures compares with the expenditures of comparable organizations. Though one must be careful of viewing expenditure percentage data as a guide to a specific organization's decisions, the fact that such data are known means that the function is worrying about its costs and is comparing itself to others.
- Ask the help desk group if it can tell you how many trouble calls it received last month, the average time to correct the problem, and the number of repeat visits. A lack of such data indicates an organization that still struggles with service provision.

Answers to these questions provide an indication, clearly rough, of how well the IT function is being run and, to a degree, whether the aggregate IT investment is providing value. All of these questions come from commonsense management beliefs in what is involved in running an organization well and tests of IT domain knowledge.

Factors That Influence Organizational IT Asset Decisions

A variety of factors influence how organizations make choices regarding the type and level of asset investment and the manner in which they manage the asset, including organizational risk tolerance, previous experiences with IT, availability of capital, the IT inclinations of the board, and the actions of competitors. Choices are made on the basis of the organization's mechanisms for assessing value and its expectations of value realization. This section focuses on two other factors that influence asset decisions: fads in the industry and surveys involving IT issues and IT adoption.

Fads

Our industry is awash in slogans; magic phrases that imply that nirvana is close at hand and that some new technology or management technique has supernatural powers that can transform organizations and the care process.

Cynicism About Slogans. Buzzwords abound in IT promises: "E-commerce" will "disintermediate" our organization, provide "seamless connectivity" between incompatible systems, and "empower consumers" to the point where they will perform their own surgery. "Open systems" provide unparalleled interoperability between applications, allowing "plug and play" that rivals Lego sets. "Application service providers" allow an organization to get deep, reliable applications at close to zero cost, enabling "reengineering" and "organizational transformation." "Data mining" will allow us to discover relationships between data that will open up new and insightful understandings about how the world works—for example, there is a correlation between light blue scrub laundry bills and surgery volume.

"Total quality management" ("TQM") will lead us all to an organization with all staff mumbling "Have a nice day" to customers and an organization that develops mission statements before it determines where to have lunch.

Slogan Tips. OK, I'm being cynical—perhaps too cynical. But at times the industry is not cynical enough. We do a disservice to our organizations, ourselves, and our professions by embracing slogans and buzzwords too quickly, especially when they are presented as having the ability to be major contributors to our asset strategies and leveraging IT's ability to further organizational strategies. A couple of thoughts and guidelines should help preserve a balance between cynicism and a too ready acceptance of fantasy.

Behind each of these slogans are pearls of truth, insight, and advancement. The pearls may be wrapped in tons of nonsense, but they are there nonetheless:

- Using rigorous analytical techniques to assess and improve core processes is critical.
- Application service providers can be a useful source of applications.
- The empowered consumer is an environmental factor that must be thoughtfully assessed.

Thus one should not dismiss slogans out of hand but rather look for pearls in them. Having found the pearls, one then needs to determine whether implementation of the nuggets of wisdom has succeeded at encapsulating the essence of the insight.

In the process of identifying the pearls, keep in the back of your mind that you have to be able to explain what you find to others. These others are usually organization board members, senior management, and medical staff. A great test of your ability to explain is if you can present it to your spouse or significant other in five minutes so that the other person understands what you have said and has not lapsed into a coma.

As you construct your explanation, you have to be able to cover the following areas:

- The root or fundamental concepts behind the pearls. For example, fundamental concepts behind TQM are that we should focus on organizational processes, be able to describe and measure them, continuously try to make them better (where better is defined by the customers of that process), and measure whether our intended improvements have actually happened.

- How the concepts and the specific implementations of these concepts will solve current problems or allow us to pursue new opportunities. In other words, why should we care if we do it at all? For example, what issues confronting a provider organization will the Web or message-based architectures solve? The answer, for some organizations, may be "not many of the important issues." This is a reasonable conclusion that would cause you to lose interest in the slogan.

- The major steps that are required if the organization wishes to pursue the pearls and their implementation. In other words, how do we capitalize on the pearls? One needs to be sure that the implementation can be grasped and is viewed as tractable and manageable.

- How to "sell" the ideas. Why would people get excited by the idea and view the steps as a reasonable series of activities to undertake in order to pursue this direction? For example, can I envision how I would get the vice president of managed care excited about the movement to XML? Selling requires that you master the three areas already listed and also that you understand your audience and what makes it tick.

- Hurdles, barriers, and risks that will confront the organization as it pursues the pearls. Failing is low on our list of things to do on any given day. One owes the organization an honest appraisal of hurdles, barriers, and risks so that it can judge whether the rewards are commensurate with the impending effort and possibility of failure. In addition to describing potential problems, one should also determine if there are strategies that can reduce their likelihood and severity.

Critical thinking is an essential component of moving from pearl identification to an effort, if warranted, to move the organization to adopt the new concepts. The thinking needs to be applied, often iteratively and with multiple contributors, in each of the areas listed.

If you cannot explain it well, you should abandon the slogan. The problem may be that you are not a very good communicator but the slogan has real merit. It doesn't matter. You won't be able to get the organization to embrace the initiative.

At times you may walk away from conferences or the reading of industry publications believing that you and your organization are the only people who have not adopted and implemented the slogan. Moreover, everyone appears to be brilliantly successful at implementing the slogan except *you*.

Don't be deceived. This work is hard and fraught with problems, and everyone has failures and partial successes. You have lots of company. Learn from the successes of others and be pleased for them. Also recognize that people tend to gloss over difficulties; they find it hard to talk about failures, and slogan enthusiasm often clouds pragmatic judgment. Also recognize that conferences and publications can only carry a small percentage of the experiences of the industry as a whole and, since they thrive on news, tend to highlight people trying new ideas; conferences and publications are not always representative of what is going on throughout the industry.

Each of these slogans, and we'll encounter many more throughout our careers, has a "life cycle" or "hype cycle." Figure 3.14 presents the cycle curve developed by the GartnerGroup (now Gartner, Inc.) that depicts various technologies at different stages of "slogan-ness." Conference hot topics and publication column inch reflect the coming and going of slogans. We should recognize that slogans and technologies have a curve.

In the beginning, some folks realize that for monetary, organizational, or academic reasons, they are on to something. Word spreads and enthusiasm builds, usually to a degree that is unwarranted. Often the original idea and its value become transformed into something that resembles the original idea but has accrued some magical properties along the way, for example, the gap between slogans that sometimes surround relational database technology today and the original Codd and Date work on the relational calculus. At other times the idea is sound but the implementations of it are neophytes, as yet unshaped by the realities of use.

People, excited by the slogan, begin to try to implement the idea. Sometimes those who try have been thoughtful about why they are doing so. Sometimes they are not. As real experience begins to accumulate, enthusiasm is replaced by a pragmatic understanding of the real value of the pearl and the challenges of imple-

FIGURE 3.14. HEALTH CARE IT HYPE CYCLE, 2001.

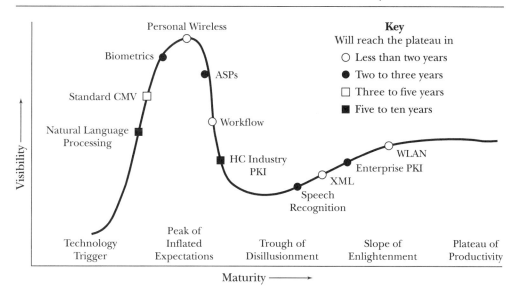

Source: Courtesy of Gartner Inc.

menting it. In addition, the developers of the technology, obtaining feedback for those who have adopted it, improve the technology, which leads to greater acceptance. Finally, we settle into a mature understanding of slogans, pearls, and their implementations.

One should realize that this curve exists. One should recognize the following points:

- Original ideas can become twisted in the early stages, at times intentionally, at times due to poor understanding of the original idea, and at times because it isn't clear to anyone whether this is an idea that should flourish or disappear.
- Early enthusiasm is often unwarranted.
- Reality will set in.
- Although one can be cynical during the early stages of this curve, one should also realize that there is likely to be real value accrued to the industry and its players.

At the end of the curve, we are better off. Cynicism should not lead to unwarranted blanket rejection of the slogan because there are pearls and the pearls will get implemented successfully by some set of people and organizations.

Surveys of Issues and IT Adoption

Surveys are regularly conducted on top IT issues in health care and across industries. Major cross-industry surveys include those conducted by Computer Science Corporation (CSC) and the Society for Information Management at the Management Information Research Center at the University of Minnesota. Examples of health care IT surveys include those conducted by the Healthcare Information and Management Systems Society (HIMSS) and Dorenfest Associates.

Survey results are often reported widely in the trade press and repackaged for presentation for internal IT discussions. Surveys do influence IT strategy and asset discussions and decisions.

These surveys are interesting and can even be useful. However, one should always be careful with the use of "normative" survey results or industry data.

The average experience or sense of priorities does not necessarily reflect the experiences and priorities of an individual organization. Being different is not equivalent to being inferior or superior or wrong or right. Nor is being average an indication of being right.

Methodological Limitations. Survey readers are often unaware of survey methodological weaknesses or approaches. The HIMSS survey captures data from a set of individuals who attend the HIMSS annual conference. Fifty percent of the HIMSS respondents are senior IT managers, and a large percentage are not. The survey cannot claim to be based on a representative sample of health care IT leaders.

Several surveys of IT issues facing provider organizations group all integrated delivery systems as one class of respondents. However, the issues facing large, geographically dispersed delivery systems can be different from those faced by a delivery system composed of a hospital and a physicians' organization. Implementing certain types of applications, such as enterprisewide scheduling, is more tractable in smaller organizations.

Some surveys, including the CSC survey, combine the results for all health care organizations. This combination would analyze, together, the responses of providers, payers, and pharmaceutical companies. These kinds of organizations face similar issues at one level—for example, appropriate use of the Internet— but dissimilar issues at another level—for example, connecting suppliers, customers, and partners electronically.

Methodological limitations can significantly limit the relevance of the results to a specific organization.

Transient Issues. Fads or new phenomena often receive very high rankings in surveys of top management issues or IT priorities. This ranking can be a reflection of anxiety about a topic or can serve as a reasonable proxy for the amount of industry buzz. However, the ranking should not necessarily be interpreted by organizational leaders as an indicator of the importance of the issue for the organization. The HIMSS 2001 survey cites "upgrading security to comply with HIPAA" as the number one IT priority. It is hard to imagine thousands of provider trustees agreeing with this assessment.

Transient issues tend to have short lives. The buzz fades, being replaced by a more pragmatic and less elevated understanding of the issue. Client-server systems were as a high-priority health care IT issue in the HIMSS surveys in 1996 and 1997 and then disappeared.

Emergent Issues. Data from surveys, such as CSC's, note which issues are trending up or down in ranking. Whenever an issue's rank changes by more than five positions over the course of several years, it would seem prudent to ask what is going on. Something is being detected by enough organizations that the phenomenon bears examination.

A decline in ranking should not indicate that an issue has become irrelevant; for example, the CSC survey noted that "cutting I/S costs" had declined to a rank of 13 in 1997 from second place in 1990. Examining and managing IT costs will always be and should always be an important issue.

Summary

Chapter Two was concerned with strategy formulation. We discussed the process of aligning organizational strategies with IT initiatives and lessons learned from decades of experiences, across a range of industries, in the application of IT to improve the competitive position of the organization. In this chapter, we were concerned with the implementation aspect of strategy and came to a number of important conclusions.

Organizations need to develop a robust, efficient, and effective IT asset. This asset consists of applications, technical architecture, data, IT staff, and IT governance. Strategies and plans are needed to ensure that the asset is and remains healthy and evolves appropriately. Ignoring the asset, or undermanaging and underfunding it, weakens the ability of the organization to effect its strategic IT plans.

Several studies of IT effectiveness have identified a relatively small number of IT-centric organizational attributes that have a significant influence on effectiveness. These attributes, bringing together much of what has been discussed in Chapters Two and Three, include the following:

- Effective means to develop IT and organizational alignment
- A focus on organizational processes, data, and differentiation
- A strong IT asset
- Thoughtful means to evaluate proposed initiatives

In addition the studies noted the importance of the following:

- IT and organizational relationships
- Senior leadership
- Organizational experience and satisfaction in working with IT

Several factors can dilute or hinder an organization's effort to realize value from its IT investments. These factors include failures to state goals, asking the wrong questions, leaping to inappropriate solutions, and mangling the management of the project. Achieving value requires management action and discipline.

Organizations should be wary of fads, slogans, and surveys that can mislead as often as they provide insight. These sources of information should not unduly influence decisions regarding strategies and changes in assets. Nor should organizations be overly cynical about what can appear to be shallowness in these sources of information.

In the next chapter, we discuss several examples, drawn from the experiences and plans of Partners HealthCare System, of the strategic application of information technology in health care. These examples will depict the alignment of organizational strategies to IT plans and the development of the related IT asset. Chapter Four will also discuss the ideas of "foundational concepts" and "strategic views."

CHAPTER FOUR

EXAMPLES OF IT STRATEGY

In this chapter, we discuss three examples of IT strategy: clinical information systems, integration, and the Internet. These examples have been drawn from strategies developed at Partners HealthCare System, Inc. During our discussion, you will witness the formulation and implementation components of strategy, the linkage of IT to the strategies of the organization, the leveraging of core organizational processes, and the development and alteration of the IT asset. These examples should serve to tie together much of the conversation in the book so far.

Each of the three examples starts from a very different premise or basic presentation of the problem or opportunity:

- Clinical information systems are an IT response directed to improving the essential capability of the provider organization: the provision of medical care. As such, clinical information systems are an example of a set of IT activities that are directly derivable from organizational strategies, plans, and competitive activities.

Notes: Portions of this chapter originally appeared in J. Glaser, "Integration of Information Systems at Partners HealthCare System," *MD Computing,* 2000, *17*(5), 23–28. Reprinted with permission.

Portions of this chapter originally appeared in J. Glaser, "The Challenge of Integrating Clinical Information systems in an Integrated Delivery System," *Topics in Health Information Management,* 1998, *19*(1), 72–77. © 1997 Aspen Publications. Reprinted with permission.

Portions of this chapter originally appeared in J. Glaser, "Management Response to the E-Health Revolution," *Frontiers in Health Services Management,* 2000, *17*(1), 45-48. Reprinted with permission.

• The integration of very heterogeneous applications and technologies is the fundamental technical challenge confronting the IDS. A parallel challenge is the creation of an IDS-wide integrated clinical system. Integration generally doesn't result from a single aspect of IDS strategy. Rather it is a necessary IT asset characteristic to support, as a foundation, a significant set of strategies of the IDS.

• The Internet, unlike clinical information systems and integration, does not fall naturally from IDS strategies. It is hard to imagine an IDS strategic discussion concluding that "we need a thing like the Internet if this core initiative is to succeed." Nor is the utility of the Internet as a component of the organization's IT asset well understood. An organization can develop a home page and provide consumer-directed health information on an intranet, but those activities, while good ideas, seem a pale use of the power of the Internet. Rather the Internet is fundamentally a profoundly social technology: its technology is not nearly as remarkable as its impact on society. In this case, the IDS challenge is to understand the role of this technology and to determine which strategies and organizational activities the technology can leverage, if any. The Internet is an example of a technology looking for a strategic fit.

In addition to discussing these examples, this chapter will focus on the development of the concepts, ideas, and definitions that govern how we view a particular IT challenge or opportunity. The importance of foundational concepts and view can be found in all aspects of our lives, and the ramifications of different views are significant. Look at some examples:

• One can view the Bible as literal, allegorical, or unverifiable and hence irrelevant.
• One can view the role of the federal government as the protector of security and individual freedoms or as a force to compensate and overcome injustice and deficiencies in the free market.
• One can view one's destiny as being heavily influenced by one's environment and one's genes, largely determined by the choices one makes in life, or preordained by larger forces in the universe.
• One can view the goal of a college education as preparation for a job, the garnering of knowledge of one's society and civilization, or an opportunity to learn how to party.

Relevant to IT, the Internet can be viewed as a means to disseminate information to patients, a mechanism to integrate heterogeneous systems, an approach to electronically moving transactions between organizations, or a catalyst for organizational transformation. These different views can lead to very different IT initiatives.

There is no one formula or recipe for arriving at a strategic view. The strategic planning frameworks discussed in Chapter Two begin with a strategic view; for example, the value chain and the competitive forces are different views of the world to be used as the basis for strategy. This chapter will not attempt to present a methodology for view development. Views emerge from complex and not well understood phenomena involving insight, discussions between members of the organization's leadership, examination of the strategic efforts of others, an organization's successes and failures (and the reasons it assigns for success and failure), and the organizational values and history that form the basis for judging views. Despite the lack of methodology in this chapter, the basis for view formation is a small number of questions. The questions are often easy to state. Developing thoughtful and insightful answers is much more difficult. Nonetheless, forming such views is critical.

This chapter, through its discussion of the three examples, presents some of the basic questions and, for three areas, answers them in an attempt to show what such views look like.

Clinical Information Systems

A portion of the conversation—the part that links IT initiatives to overall strategic initiatives and plans—is conceptually straightforward. For example, if the organization intends to manage physician practices, there will be a need for application systems that support the related administrative operations of billing and scheduling. If the organization intends to improve its abilities to measure the quality of its care, there will be a need for appropriate databases and analytical tools. While the mapping of strategy to IT response may be clear, the implementation of the response may be quite complex and difficult.

A portion of the conversation is more conceptually complex. The strategy implies (or is explicit about) deep changes in the organization and significant changes in the nature of the application systems. For example, an HMO moving from a staff model, where physicians are salaried, to a model where its physicians are paid for performance will undergo deep organizational change. The application systems needed to support performance measurement are also likely to represent a significant change in the current application portfolio and the data of the HMO. The implementation will be difficult because of these factors.

Several questions should be asked as the organization examines its strategies and the linkage to IT activities.

Does the strategy imply that there are new and significant concepts that govern how we organize, practice, incentivize, or structure the work? There are many examples of strategies that would answer in the affirmative:

- An effort to decentralize decision making at a provider organization with a national presence
- A strategy to aggressively pursue risk sharing and assume as much medical management as possible
- An effort to move as many patients as possible to protocol-driven care
- A strategy to develop a continuum of care

What are the underlying concepts behind these strategies?

- An effort to assume a significant amount of risk can represent the concept that the provider organization will engage in the full spectrum of medical management believing that it can do it better, and for less money, than managed care organizations and improve its leverage over managed care organizations and employers.
- The development of a continuum of care can represent a concept that purchasers of care will want to deal with one provider organization for all of their care needs. In addition, the provider will be able to rationalize care across the continuum, leading to cost reductions and service and care quality improvements.

Does the IT response represent new concepts for applications, architecture, or any other part of the asset? What are the concepts?

- A continuum of care, if it involves linking a wide range of diverse clinical information systems, may require that the concepts and techniques behind the integration of systems become far more robust and diverse.
- The movement to protocol-driven care may require that clinical information systems and clinical support systems like scheduling have deep and powerful capabilities to add and integrate algorithms, perform complex logic checks, and integrate pathway development into existing applications.

Applications that are based on new concepts are inherently risky to implement. What are the risk factors that will accompany the IT response, and what strategies and steps are available to overcome the risks? The organizational risks may not involve the IT group or the technology; for example, a provider organization assuming risk may face its greatest peril in the HMO competitive response or the organization getting into a line of business in which it has little experience. The IT group or the technology may be the focal point of risk—for example, can today's integration technologies provide the desired integration between heterogeneous platforms and applications? Or are needed clinical information systems designed in a way that fits well into physician workflow?

In this section, we will focus on clinical information systems. These systems are an example of an application portfolio and agenda that can be derived directly from the organization's strategies. They are also an example of an area where there is often significant change in the underlying concepts of both the business and the applications, and hence organizational and IT risk are involved.

Core Business Concepts and Views

Health care providers face several significant cost, quality, and access pressures on care delivery. To meet these pressures, they must, with increasing sophistication and effectiveness, do all of the following:

- Measure and report the quality of care outcomes and processes
- Identify and manage "optimal" medical care processes
- Streamline or redesign care-related operations
- Reduce the cost of care per unit, per encounter, and per covered life
- Improve customer satisfaction

In their efforts to respond to these pressures, the organization may realize that there are two major concepts that will guide the response to these pressures. Both concepts must be refined before being implemented.

The first concept is an increased emphasis on organizational clinical management of care. Care processes and outcomes can be measured, best practices can be defined and implemented, and conformance to these practices can be monitored. These practices can be applied, by the organization, to specific care acts—for example, encouraging providers to use cheaper, therapeutically equivalent medications. The practices can be applied to an encounter, such as a clinical pathway for coronary arterial bypass graft surgery. And the practices can be applied to care that spans encounters—for example, guidelines for the treatment of hypertension.

The second concept is that care should be viewed as a process: a series of interdependent tasks and activities performed by a diverse set of health care professionals and the patient. The process can be analyzed, measured, and reengineered. These activities span providers, departments, organizations, and time. The view of care as a process is different from the view of care in terms of discrete knowledge domains, such as oncology, or in terms of departments and roles, such as nursing or the clinical laboratories.

IT Application Concepts

The focus of clinical information systems should be the support of organizational efforts to implement its definition of these two approaches. Clinical information systems are the application systems used by providers to support the immediate provision of care. Examples include the computerized patient record, provider order entry, and databases that are used to measure care quality.

Three major goals for clinical information systems can be stated:

- To improve the efficiency and effectiveness of care-centric processes. Examples include accessing data about a patient, ordering something, and referring a patient. Information systems should make these processes less error-prone, less expensive, faster, and more convenient.
- To improve provider and patient decision making. In their efforts to implement best-care practices, organizations would like to ensure that as decisions are made, the most appropriate decisions are reached. These decisions can range from ordering the most appropriate radiology modality given the clinical question to defining the right care activities on postoperative day 2 for a specific procedure to the best diet for someone with high cholesterol. At times the objective is to prevent an adverse decision, for example, the ordering of a medication to which the patient is allergic. If the organization has no position on the "best" decision, it can offer knowledge resources, for example, medical textbooks, guidelines developed by professional societies, or literature-searching capabilities.
- To evaluate the efficiency and effectiveness of care. Databases and analysis capabilities should be provided to enable the organization to understand its care practices, identify optimal practices, monitor its conformance to those practices, and report its outcomes and measures of care processes to a variety of constituencies.

Drawing from the discussion of concepts and goals, the view of clinical information systems can be stated in the form of philosophies and concepts that guide clinical information systems activities and plans.

The broad objective is care process improvement. This statement is seemingly self-evident. However, it suggests that one deduces the applications and application capabilities needed from a thorough analysis of care process problems and opportunities for improvement. The organization should not leap to the conclusion that it needs computerized records or any other application until it is sure that it has developed an understanding of the care problems to be solved and the specific linkages between application capabilities and problem reduction or removal are very clear.

An important IT concept is the "information-rich" process. Most clinical decisions are made in the context of a process; for example, the decision to refer initiates the referral process, and the decision to order a medication initiates the ordering process. Information systems directed to improving the process have an opportunity to deliver information or check decisions at key points in the process.

For example, the application, while capturing clinical data to be transmitted to the consulting physician, can check to see if the referral is being directed to the right specialist or is even necessary. As medications are ordered, the system can check for allergies, contraindications, and opportunities to suggest less expensive therapeutic equivalents.

There are a relatively small number of core care processes. Perhaps the use of the word *core* makes the adjective *small* self-fulfilling. Nonetheless, for example, the application of IT should focus on accessing clinical data, ordering, and referring a patient for an admission or to a specialist. It is with these processes that the IT application system response must be "A-plus."

Process leverage points are poorly understood. Our knowledge of how best to apply IT to improve care is crude. There is insufficient industry experience with these systems and insufficient measurement of experiences where they have occurred. We have much to learn. Hence clinical information systems must be designed in a way such that the systems can continuously and efficiently be changed to respond to improved knowledge about the care process.

The use of IT to improve care is a form of guerrilla war. There is no single application system, no core set of capabilities, no single database that once installed will turn the tide in the battle to improve care. Care is too complex. There are no decisive battles here. Rather care improvement is a year-in, year-out, continuous set of initiatives: a form of guerrilla war. Wars can be won this way.

The implementation of clinical information systems is a countless-project journey that has no end. Advances in basic science, medical practice, pharmaceuticals, and diagnostic technologies will mean that no matter how advanced our medical practice is, it will always be able to be better. Hence no matter what capabilities our clinical systems have, there will be care improvement opportunities. We will never be done in our efforts to apply IT to improving medical care. Defining and building the ultimate clinical information system is a wasteful exercise in that it implies that we know the end point and that there is an end point.

Organizations should focus. Organizations should be wary of blanket statements about the need to make care paperless or to "fully automate the medical record." Instead, for any given year, there should be a set of well-defined initiatives that have several characteristics:

• They solve very clear, measurable care problems or provide opportunities to improve care.
• They focus on processes comprehensively.
• They use applications that are developed and implemented within an overall clinical information systems architecture (look back at Figure 3.2 for an example).
• They leverage an IT ability to support the iterative improvement in care.

This wariness does not mean that the computerization of the record is a bad idea. Rather it is a recognition that the computerization of the record becomes a by-product of efforts to improve care practices, almost a secondary outcome, instead of being the primary objective.

Sources of Complexity

The design and implementation of clinical information systems has always been complex. Three major factors or sources have contributed most of the complexity: the process of care, health and medical data, and care boundaries. These sources create challenges that are in addition to challenges, which occur at times, posed by new technology that doesn't work as advertised, recalcitrant providers, and organizational confusion.

Before the advent of the IDS, these challenges existed. However, the creation of integrated delivery systems, an increasingly stringent reimbursement environment, and demands for more accountability for the cost effectiveness of care have led to pressures that have aggravated the complexities. For example, the industry is adding to its traditional challenge of integrating departmental systems the challenge of integrating systems across organizations. The industry's interest in implementing clinical systems is moving beyond traditional hospital-centric systems to systems that support a continuum of care. And although the cost of care will always be a basis of competition, quality, and proving quality, is ascending in importance to the purchaser of care.

These sources of complexity have a significant impact on the difficulty of implementing clinical systems and are unlikely to be resolved in the immediate future.

Complexity of the Process of Care. If one were to view the process of care as a manufacturing process (sick people as inputs, a "bunch of stuff" is done to them, and better or well people emerge), it is arguable that medical care is the most complex manufacturing process that exists. This type of complexity has three major sources: defining best care, process variability, and process volatility.

Our current ability to define the best care process for treating a particular disease or problem can be limited. Process algorithms, guidelines, or pathways are often based on heuristics that makes consensus within and between organizations difficult or impossible. Factual or scientific evidence that can act as the final arbitrator leading to a consistent effective approach is often insufficient. We often arrive at competing guidelines or protocols being issued by payers, provider organization committees, and provider associations.

Process guidelines are also often specific to the condition or context. The treatment of a particular acute illness, for example, can depend on the severity of the illness and the age and general health of the patient. Guidelines are also often reliant on outcome measurements that can have severe limitations; for example, they can be insensitive to specific interventions, serve as proxies for true outcomes, or reflect the bias of the organization or the researcher.

Many an organization has failed to define and apply a consistent approach to care. But even a defined approach may permit substantial latitude on the part of the provider. Consequently, treatment can be subject to great variability. In an academic medical center, a physician may be able to order one of 2,500 medications (each with a set of "allowable" frequencies, doses, and routes), 1,100 clinical laboratory tests, 300 radiology procedures, and large numbers of other tests and procedures. The sequence and time relationship, along with patient condition and comorbidity, all determine the relative utility of a particular approach to treatment. The variability within approaches to treating a disease is compounded by the diversity of disease and problems. There are 10,000 diseases, each of which, in theory, has a different pathway, guideline, or approach.

This variability, or opportunity for variability, is unparalleled by any other manufacturing process. No automobile manufacturer produces 10,000 different models of cars or provides, for each model, 2,500 different types of paint, 300 different arrangements of wheels, or 1,100 different locations for the driver's seat.

If we presumed that through hard work and a very agreeable group of providers, we finally develop a large number of guidelines and algorithms and had significantly reduced the options in test, medication, and procedure ordering, we would be confronted with the volatility of the medical process. In an average year, sixty thousand articles are added to the base of refereed medical literature, which may lead us to need to continuously revisit our consensus. In addition, medical technology often induces us to change practices before the studies that measure their efficacy can be completed.

The complexity of the medical process places unique and tough demands on the design of clinical information systems, our ability to support provider and patient decision making, and our ability to measure the quality of the care that we deliver. It is a complex undertaking to rationalize or standardize these processes within one provider organization. Clearly, we compound the problem as we move across organizations within an IDS and from there expand beyond the IDS boundaries. We may end up attempting to have application systems interoperate in support of different approaches to care.

Complexity of Health and Medical Data. The health status and medical condition of a patient is difficult to describe using comprehensive, coded data. Factors that contribute to this problem include the following:

- Although research is ongoing, accepted methods for formally decomposing many key components of the patient record, such as admission history and physical, into coded concepts have not yet been developed.
- Even when such data models have been developed, vocabularies to represent the terms within the model in a standard way are difficult to develop. The condition of a patient is often complex, probabilistic, and highly nuanced. Multifactorial and temporal relationships can exist between pieces of data. This complexity makes it inherently difficult to develop codes for medical data.
- Even when the model has been developed and coded terms have been defined, entry of coded data, by the provider, is more cumbersome and constraining than using free text.
- Finally, several additional factors contribute to the complexity of data. There is no single way to organize automated medical data. The relational model does not serve the medical domain particularly well. And one encounters, across sites and often within a site, idiosyncratic ways to code data that have often been developed for good reasons, and because of the significant investments made to define and implement this approach, change will not happen unless it is very compelling.

Because coding schemes can be idiosyncratic, nonexistent, or insufficient within and across organizations in an IDS, establishing clinical meaning, measuring care, determining the health status of a patient, and developing clinical information systems that interoperate can be exquisitely difficult.

Complexity of Care Boundaries. An organizational boundary—for example, the physician groups, hospitals, and subacute facilities that make up an IDS—does not adequately bound the patterns of health care encounters experienced by people considered to be members of the organization. A person may receive care at hospitals or physician offices that are part of the IDS. That person may also receive care in settings outside the IDS, or data about patients may be generated by organizations outside the IDS, as in the case of a retail pharmacy.

If the IDS desires to create a composite clinical picture of a person, as through the implementation of a clinical data repository, it needs clinical data from multiple care settings, some of which are part of the IDS and some of which are not. The IDS may decide that it needs applications to span all of these settings; for example, it may need to have a computerized record in all of these settings or at least have these records interoperate. The complexity created by this "leakiness" or "blurriness" in organizational boundaries shows up in several ways.

Thousands or millions of people, who an IDS considers to be its membership, may receive care, in aggregate, in potentially dozens or hundreds of settings that are not part of the IDS. An IDS may decide to connect its systems to these other settings. The connection could be in the form of providing access to IDS applications, through a workstation or Web access, at these settings. The resulting pattern of system interconnections, when carried out over a region or a state by multiple provider organizations, is a complex network topology model, with almost every provider connected to every other provider.

We complicate this pattern by "random" dispersion of data. One site, despite having a clinical data repository, may need to access data being kept at other sites. But the requesting site may not know where these data exist or if they exist or whether the data are relevant. One may not know, for a patient who presents at the emergency room, whether the patient has been seen in other hospitals in the city.

Should we be able to effect this "interconnectedness" and do so efficiently, we would still have to grapple with the complexity created by the fact that we often want to do more than provide access to applications across these sites. We want to exchange data and have application processes interoperate. However, we see, across settings, significant variations in data, clinical processes, definitions of optimal processes, and the extant base of information systems:

- Data definitions vary across settings. These variations exist in problem lists, laboratory tests, procedures, and other types of clinical data.
- Care processes vary. Referrals, medication ordering, care documentation, and other processes are not done the same way across settings.
- Definitions of optimal care vary. Frequency of visits, standard batteries of tests, and appropriate medications for a particular problem are not consistent across settings.
- One will clearly encounter different technologies, vendors, and levels of IT sophistication across settings. One will also find different levels of computerization; for example, some settings will have provider order entry while others will not.

The nature of the relationships between organizations, both within the IDS and across its boundaries, will change over time. Hospitals in the IDS may decide to consolidate to one microbiology laboratory but leave other parts of the clinical laboratory unintegrated. A provider and a payer may decide that both organizations need not do utilization review and decide to integrate that function between them.

An integrated delivery system, if it desires to have a comprehensive database about the health status and care received by one of its members or have clinical applications interoperate, faces a daunting challenge due to the fact that care is often boundaryless. The complexity of boundaries compounds the complexities of the medical process and health and medical data.

Brigham and Women's Hospital Care Improvement Efforts

We shall now discuss a specific effort of Brigham and Women's Hospital (BWH) to apply IT to improve the process of care in the interest of reducing adverse drug events. This effort, discussed in depth elsewhere (Teich and others, 1996), is illustrative of several of the concepts discussed in this chapter:

- Medical care was examined as a process, with studies identifying deficiencies in the process.
- Information system capabilities were derived as a result of understanding process failure points.
- The studies highlighted the need to have information systems support an information-rich process (the core view of the IT response), specifically, provider order entry with decision support. An information process is one that is "aware" of what the task performer is trying to do and provides information, as needed, to guide the actions of the task performer. For example, the process is aware that the physician is trying to order a medication that is contraindicated and provides information that points out the problem and suggests alternative actions.
- The order entry system required that some (but not all) aspects of care complexity be addressed. Aspects addressed included the codification of allergies and medications, the pursuit of one process (provider decision making), and the process as it occurs for inpatients (establishing an inpatient boundary).
- The application had to possess a high degree of agility—for example, a set of tools to allow efficient construction of order sets—so that the system could respond efficiently to the progressive understanding of the care process and its opportunities for improvement (application system strategy).
- The efforts involved change or development of several other aspects of the IT asset: infrastructure, data, governance, and IT staff.

Adverse Drug Event Reduction at BWH. A team led by Leape and Bates (Leape and others, 1995; Bates and others, 1994) examined the incidence and nature of adverse drug events at Brigham and Women's Hospital (BWH) and Massachusetts General Hospital (MGH). The study's findings:

- 6.5 adverse drug events (ADEs) occurred per 100 non-OB admissions, an estimated 2,340 annually at BWH.
- 28 percent of ADEs, or 655 ADEs, were preventable.
- 5.5 potential ADEs occur per 100 non-OB admissions, an estimated 1,980 annually for BWH. These errors, such as the order for a medication that was contraindicated, did not result in an event because they were caught by a nurse or pharmacist before execution of the order was complete.
- The average cost of each ADE was $6,000.

The ADE problem was clearly significant. Further analysis examined the nature of the IT solution (Bates and others, 1994):

- 56 percent of the ADEs occur at time of ordering: the physician is unaware of or forgets about an allergy, a contraindication, or a problematic laboratory result.
- 34 percent of the ADEs occur at time of medication administration, with some of these being due to order legibility problems.
- For BWH, a provider order entry system could prevent an estimated 480 ADEs per year, for an annual savings of $2.9 million. This system would need to have the following capabilities:
  Drug interaction checking
  Drug-lab checking
  Drug allergy checking
  Drug dosing based on age and renal status
  Informational displays of current results

The ADE study clearly pointed to the need for a provider order entry system. For maximum reduction of ADEs, the system would have to be used by the ordering physician for the entry of all medication orders.

An internal BWH study examined the ordering of six common laboratory tests in the surgical intensive care unit (ICU). The study concluded that 35 to 50 percent of the tests were clinically unnecessary, often the result of "preprogrammed" ordering—for example, an order for routine blood tests four times a day for four days. A provider order entry system could also reduce problems of inappropriate test ordering if entry were expanded to include all orders by the physician. Figure 4.1 provides an example of an order entry screen. Figure 4.2 provides an example of a warning designed to reduce medication errors.

FIGURE 4.1. MEDICATION ORDER ENTRY.

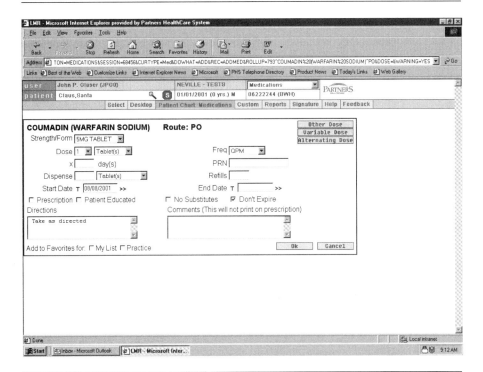

Impact on the IT Asset. An organizational decision to pursue the implementation of a provider order entry system clearly requires an investment in the application component of the IT asset: an order entry application. Not only was designing and developing a provider order entry system extremely complex, but the asset impact was more extensive than an application system.

Application utilities software are software tools that are part of the application. Examples include tools to support schedule creation and editing in an outpatient scheduling system or editing of payer dictionaries in an accounts receivable system.

The provider order entry system required several application utilities: software to process medical logic or rules, tools to enable users to construct order sets, and tools to link order screens to knowledge resources.

The infrastructure required upgrading primarily to ensure very high degrees of reliability and significantly enhanced potency. Downtime for an order entry system is highly problematic, particularly if there is no corresponding paper copy

FIGURE 4.2. MEDICATION ALLERGY WARNING.

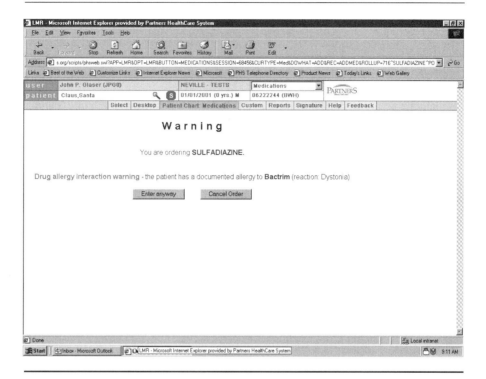

of the orders. If a results reporting system fails, the provider can call the laboratory; there are fewer practical options when order entry downtime occurs.

Upon entering an order, the system would engage in a series of checks to ensure that the order was safe and did not represent a potentially inappropriate consumption of resources. Several dozen rules might be invoked for each order, and these rules had to check potentially dozens of pieces of data. Because most orders will be acceptable, this checking process has to be exceptionally fast, since few providers want to wait more than a second only to be told that their order was "correct." Hence order entry had to be assisted by very fast processing power and data access. These potency needs, and others, led BWH to implement a very large client-server platform (Roberts, 1995).

Organizational data and databases required progress in two major areas. First, order-checking logic meant that coded allergies and reasons for an order had to be established and implemented. Vocabularies for medications, procedures, and laboratory tests and associated results had to be reviewed and augmented.

Second, a database of orders and related clinical information was to be created from the order transactions. This database would allow BWH to assess its ordering patterns and outcomes on an ongoing basis.

Three major categories of IT staff had to be defined, organized, and hired to support this and other similar systems.

Medical informatics talent was hired to provide the domain knowledge and effort to develop medical logic processors, define vocabularies for data to be coded, work with the medical staff to analyze and design care interventions, and lead the design of the order entry system such that it fit well with clinical workflow and thought processes.

IT staff were needed who could perform the implementation tasks associated with clinical information systems that have a deep impact on care operations and processes. These staff had to analyze and possibly reengineer workflows, train clinicians, provide front-line support during implementation, and manage specification development for suggested enhancements. These staff were predominantly people who had clinical backgrounds, particularly in nursing.

Care management analysis talent, who had health services research training, were recruited to support ongoing analyses of care processes and to measure the impact of the order entry system and other clinical information systems to determine if the desired improvements in care occurred following system implementation.

IT governance was altered in two major ways. First, the overall guidance for clinical information systems, beginning with the provider order entry system, was placed under the jurisdiction of existing BWH care quality improvement forums. The BWH Care Improvement Steering Committee (CISC), composed of senior clinical and administrative leaders (including the BWH CIO), had been formed to provide overall direction, policy setting, and resource allocation for efforts designed to improve care operations and practices. In addition to order entry guidance, for example, this committee initiated the development of clinical pathways. The Clinical Initiatives Committee (CIC), reporting to the CISC, had been formed to identify and prioritize the care processes and areas that would be assessed for opportunities for improvement, develop improvement plans, and monitor progress. Members of the medical informatics and care management analysis staff were on the CIC.

Knowledge domain committees were established, and existing committees had their role expanded. The Pharmacy and Therapeutics Committee was tapped, and laboratory and radiology utilization committees were formed to perform the following functions:

- Provide ongoing review and definition of new logic to be applied in an effort to reduce adverse events and improve utilization

- Ensure that the logic was defensible, on the basis of the literature or the consensus of the committee's medical expertise
- Ensure that the medical staff were informed of the rationale for the logic
- Monitor the impact of the logic on care practice
- Update the logic as advances in medical practice occurred
- Respond to questions about the logic and its clinical rationale

The diagram in Figure 4.3 illustrates the broad IT asset impact of clinical information systems.

Strategies Surrounding Implementation. We haven't yet discussed strategies that might surround the implementation of a specific system. In Chapter One, implementation was defined, broadly, as an element of strategy. Implementation strategies have been discussed in the context of the organization being structured, resourced, and organized such that multiple application implementations can occur in ways that further the formulation component of strategy. An example of a broad implementation strategy is the creation of a group of medical informatics staff to be applied across multiple clinical systems implementations or the establishment of a highly reliable technical infrastructure to support multiple clinical systems.

Strategies surrounding the implementation of a specific application are generally designed to overcome major sources of implementation risk or address implementation critical success factors.

The BWH provider order entry system had two major critical success factors:

- Direct physician use of a complicated application that performed a critical process
- Physicians' acceptance of their clinical judgment being challenged by a computer

Strategies designed to address one factor also addressed the other. Several of these strategies will be discussed.

There is no substitute for a well-designed, easy-to-use application that "thinks" like the user. The design approaches and guidelines of the BWH provider order entry system are described by Teich and others (1995) and will not be repeated here. Let us look at some of the other physician use strategies.

- The system was developed internally. The complexity of the application meant that it was inevitable that the initial specifications were, at best, 80 percent right. The system also had a suggestion button that allowed users to forward ideas.

FIGURE 4.3. CLINICAL INFORMATION SYSTEMS IT ASSET.

Overview of Clinical Information System Infrastructure

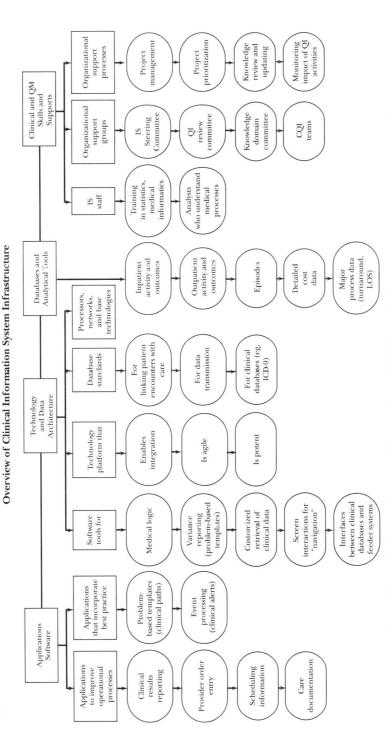

To support retrospective analysis; monitoring conformance to best practices; analysis of operational processes.

A clinical information system must encompass four key components: applications software, technology and data architecture, databases and analytical tools, and clinical and quality management (QM) skills and supports. Key: LOS = length of stay; IS = information services; CQI = continuous quality improvement; QI = quality improvement.

Source: Copyright © John P. Glaser: "The Role of the Chief Information Officer in Forming Clinical Information System Strategies." *Joint Commission Journal of Quality Improvement, 20,* 614–621, fig. 1, 1994. Reprinted with permission.

Though some of these ideas had to do with the removal of various parts of the anatomy of the IT staff, most of the ideas were helpful. IT staff were able to respond rapidly to these suggestions and enhance the system or correct bugs. The mantra was "If there are ten suggestions on Monday, six will be implemented by Friday. There will be ten on the following Monday, and four will be left on the following Friday." The system evolved rapidly, based on real experience, with its use becoming more "right" every week. This also meant that medical staff saw sustained improvement in the system and a willingness to listen to their ideas. This approach is related to the discussion, in Chapter Three, of achieving agility through the internal development of applications.

• Once implementation was started in a service, the implementation would move at "warp speed" through the service. A lull would ensue to enable staff to catch their breath, and then implementation would resume again. For example, the medicine service was implemented in four weeks. A two-month lull occurred before a six-week push through surgery. This pace of burst-lull-burst minimized the amount of time that physicians spent straddling manual and computer-based orders as they made their rounds.

• All care units were staffed with personnel around the clock for the first two weeks of the system's introduction to ensure that help was available in the form a person within eyeshot. Training classes were sparsely attended, and retention of material covered in training was poor. People will not read the manual, nor are they likely to call the number posted on the workstation. They will respond to a pleasant person coming up to them and asking if they can help. Delivery of this help early in the implementation was essential to ensuring use.

The implementation of a system that has, as its core premise, the intent to challenge the real-time decision making of the physician can appear to be threatening. Hence while this implementation, like all implementations, had to address issues of software capabilities, training, and infrastructure readiness, the implementation of provider order entry had the additional burden of developing strategies to handle the potential problems of real-time decision support.

To address this critical success factor, the following strategies were developed and implemented:

• The analyses of the incidence of adverse drug events and the use of laboratory tests in the surgery ICU provided the basis for significant political support on the part of the clinical leadership. The support was almost in the form of a moral imperative. The analyses of care deficiencies were of very high quality, conducted by physicians who were respected as health services researchers. It was difficult to attack the quality of the study or the credentials of the researchers. The data indicated a serious problem that was not only financial but also, in case of the adverse events, counter to the core medical ethos of the medical staff leadership. To a large degree, the motive to solve this problem was based on core values and not on dollars or notions of efficiency.

- The first interventions or medical logic focused on interventions that were "no brainers." It is hard to argue with the utility of a piece of logic that points out allergies or medication contraindications.

- The system was "packaged" as an experiment. It would be piloted and evaluated. It would be implemented and evaluated. If the evaluation showed that the system created more problems than it solved or failed to live up to its expectations, it would be removed. This packaging eased the sense that the system was a "given" with administration doggedly committed to implementation regardless of the consequences. This packaging also fit with the culture of BWH, an academic medical center, which was quite comfortable with the notion of conducting well-designed experiments with the intent of seeing whether the intervention improved care or not.

In addition to being labeled an experiment, other aspects of system implementation were designed to ensure that the rules were "safe":

- Resources were committed to ongoing evaluation of the impact of the system.
- Knowledge domain committees were established to ensure that the appropriate expertise was brought to the task of constructing logic.
- Rules were often introduced as a designed "experimental" trial; for example, the rules were activated for half the patients and not the other half, to ensure a trial period before full implementation.
- Computer-generated advice could be overridden by the physician (although as the system made the transition from an experiment to an accepted aspect of the clinical management of care, medical leadership became increasing comfortable with not permitting immediate overriding of some interventions).

Impact. The provider order entry system, using a core view of an information-rich process, has had a significant impact on the care at BWH (Teich and others, 1996, 2000). Here are some examples of that impact:

- On an average day, 13,000 orders were entered by a clinician, and 386 of these were changed as a result of a computer suggestion.
- Serious medication errors decreased by 55 percent (Bates and others, 1998).
- Nizatidine (the preferred H2 blocker) use increased, as a percentage of all H2 blocker orders, from 12 percent to 81 percent.

- The percentage of medication doses over the suggested maximum decreased from 2 percent to 0.6 percent.
- The percentage of orders for ondansetron, with the preferred frequency of three times daily, increased from 6 percent to 75 percent.
- The percentage of bed rest orders with a consequent order of heparin increased from 24 percent to 54 percent after the computer reminded the physician to order heparin.

Clinical Information Systems Across a Continuum of Care

When we examine the challenge of clinical information systems across a continuum of care, we find that the concepts and views developed originally for inpatient care support can be extended, although they undergo some transformation.

The two core views of clinical management of care and the perspective of care as a process remain the same. However, they are not completely the same. The focus of clinical management can change. For example, the clinical management of care over a continuum (in contrast to an encounter or a specific care act such as a medication order) has a greater emphasis on the management of the chronically ill. The relative importance of a process can change. For example, the presence of a risk arrangement may place more emphasis on streamlining the process of referrals than on inpatient procedure ordering.

Core views, if they are well conceived, tend to remain intact over long periods of time. This does not mean that they remain unaltered. However, organizational competency in the clinical management of care, for example, will serve as a strength even as the view evolves.

The three IT goals for improving care remain: improve care processes, enhance decision making, and evaluate the quality and cost of care. Nonetheless, they too undergo change. The referral becomes more important both as a means to channel patients to care settings within the system, minimizing "leakage," and to support medical management. Accessing data, always an important process, moves from a hospital-centric issue to an IDS-centric issue, leading to the creation of a clinical data repository. If an organization places great emphasis on wellness, the focus of decision-making improvements may expand.

The clinical information systems complexity factors loom larger in a continuum than in an acute care hospital. The IDS inherently spans multiple organizations, and hence the complexity of boundary spanning is exacerbated and the challenge of integration is heightened. The creation of a continuum involves collecting data on care patterns from disparate organizations within the IDS, which compounds the complexities of differences in data definitions and care processes.

The observations on the care process remain intact. Care improvement is still iterative. Organizations should still begin with process examination from which the capabilities of applications can be derived.

Problems and Opportunities in Outpatient Care and the Care Continuum. As in the adverse medication error example, the formation of clinical systems for a continuum begins with an analysis of care processes to identify their deficiencies. Internal studies at Partners of such processes generated the following data.

In a study of clinic patients (Sittig, 1998), 18 percent reported problems or unexpected symptoms after taking their medications. Nearly half (48 percent) of those with problems sought medical attention. Those who experienced problems reported lower satisfaction with their care. In essence, it appears that 9 percent of the outpatient encounters may be associated with problems with medications prescribed at a previous visit.

In a study of primary care provider (PCP) and specialist (SSP) satisfaction with the referral process, Gandhi and others (1998) revealed the following findings:

- 63 percent of the PCPs and 35 percent of the SSPs were dissatisfied with the referral process.
- PCPs reported that only 36 percent of the time did they receive a SSP follow-up within seven days.
- For 23 percent of the referrals, SSPs did not have enough information to adequately address the patient's problem.

This analysis suggested that care improvement opportunities might be extensive. A range of possible improvements is presented in Table 4.1.

Continuum IT Asset. Analyses of the data and discussions with other delivery systems and Partners' providers led to the identification of a set of applications and related features necessary to support an effective and efficient continuum of care. Moreover, changes to all aspects of the IT asset were identified as being necessary. (Strategies for the integration of clinical information systems will be discussed in the next section; the impact on the asset is discussed here.)

Applications. Several application needs were identified (Teich, 1998):

• A computerized medical record to support the documentation of care (structured according to flowsheets where appropriate), the accessibility of clinical data between providers, and the incorporation of health maintenance reminders.

TABLE 4.1. POSSIBLE CONTINUUM IMPROVEMENTS.

Objective	Clinical Information System
15 percent overall decrease in pmpm outpatient medication drug costs	Ambulatory Order Entry
50 percent decrease in inappropriateness rate for targeted tests, such as Digoxin, PSA, and thyroid function tests	Ambulatory Order Entry
15 percent net decrease in radiology use	Ambulatory Order Entry
80 percent decrease in outpatient medication errors	Ambulatory Order Entry
50 percent improvement in speed of processing of Referral Application	Referral Application
99 percent complete data for key Referral Application fields, such as diagnosis, number of visits, and who the patient is to see	Referral Application
30 percent decrease in out-of-network Referral Application	Referral Application
100 percent documentation of follow-up for abnormal Pap smears	Computerized Medical Record
70 percent vaccination rate for all eligible patients	Computerized Medical Record

• A referral application to support the comprehensive communication of data between the referring and consulting physician, provide logic to check for any referral preconditions, and determine referral necessity; establish linkages to scheduling systems to ensure that the referral was scheduled.

• Provider order entry for outpatient visits focusing on medication ordering and prescription generation but also supporting radiology and laboratory orders. Logic, similar to that used for inpatient order entry, would check the orders for safety and appropriate utilization.

In addition to improving the continuum-based processes of care, Partners' strategies also called for the extension of the clinical reach of its specialists. As the clinical management of care across a continuum becomes more important and managed care cost pressures increase, the need for efficient access to specialists is elevated. A telemedicine program was initiated to develop applications to extend the reach of the specialist throughout the region and the globe. The program also implements applications designed to improve the ability of Partners to support the remote management of the chronically ill at home. A program to support the development of Picture Archival and Communications Systems (PACS) applications was initiated. PACS applications serve to improve the accessibility of images throughout the continuum.

Clinical Information Systems Utilities. The clinical information systems utilities evolved to incorporate new demands placed by the view of care as a continuum and the heightened emphasis of clinical information systems in the ambulatory care settings. These utility elements included flowsheet templates for the gathering of structured outpatient data, guideline and algorithm development templates, and additional access restriction algorithms to protect the confidentiality of patients. Confidentiality looms as a significantly larger concern as clinical information systems grow to encompass relatively large numbers of care settings and patients.

Infrastructure. Infrastructure strategies were augmented, largely in the area of application integration, which will be discussed later in this chapter. In addition to integration, a continuum faces significant boundary problems. For both integration and boundary reasons, the technology architecture was moved to "lowest common denominator technologies," for example, TCP/IP and browser-based front ends. This term is by no means pejorative. Rather the movement recognizes that the IDS systems must be extended to, and loosely integrated with, systems in care settings in which the IDS has little or no control, such as an affiliated health center with which there is a referral arrangement. The IDS is unlikely to have much interest in expending the capital required to place a workstation on the desk of this health center or being responsible for the support of invasive applications that interfere with the client configuration adopted by the health center. And yet the IDS desires to extend its reach and to be able to do so quickly. Lowest common denominator technologies also enable IDS infrastructure to be supportable and agile.

Data. Most of the clinical data in a continuum have to be mappable to a common vocabulary. Laboratory tests can be mapped to the LOINC standard. Problems can be mapped to the ICD-9 codes. Medications can be mapped to one of several national standard dictionaries. It may be quite difficult to force extant application systems to adopt these standards, but new systems can be implemented using the standard, and the clinical data repository can have all incoming data mapped to these standards before being stored.

The construction of a database of IDS-wide quality measures will bring forth a range of data inconsistencies and quality issues. A simple quality measure such as unplanned returns to the operating room may encounter different definitions of "unplanned" and, in the various organizations, different individuals—for example, operating room nurses versus billing clerks—deciding whether the second procedure was planned or unplanned.

Staff. The IT staff asset may have to undergo some change. In the case of Partners, a small number of new IT groups were created:

- The Telemedicine Center conducts trials of the use of telemedicine to support the remote delivery of care and the extension of the specialist over a wide geographical area. The group also supports videoconferencing activity used by the integrated residency programs and also used to extend access to medical education and rounds throughout the region.
- The Data Analysis unit supports the databases and analysis of Partners-wide care quality measurement and care pattern assessment.
- The Medical Imaging group is responsible for developing PACS to support radiology and other specialty image capture, storage, and transmission and the extension of radiology services to community-based practices.

In addition, existing groups (the Medical Informatics group and those staff that developed clinical applications and implemented them) had to develop an appreciation for care practice and organizational cultures that were not academic medical center–based. The world of a two-person physician practice in rural New Hampshire and that of the suburban community hospital are not the same as that of a Harvard teaching affiliate. These differences are not instantly appreciated or understood by staff who trained in an academic medical center.

IT Governance. The guidance of clinical information system activities at Partners evolved to the following current form:

- The Partners Executive Committee, composed of the member organization CEOs and the physician leaders, provides overall direction on strategies and priorities, including IT, and approves the final budgets.
- The Partners System Integration Committee develops the enterprise strategy for the integration of patient care, research, and education. Made up of most of the Partners Executive Committee, this group reviews and approves the IT clinical integration strategy.
- Each hospital has a physician advisory group that works on issues and needs for its local physician community. These groups hold joint sessions to establish priorities and recommend directions.
- The practice medical directors, from across Partners physician practices, contribute guidance on systems issues related to primary care and medical management.

Observations and Issues. The implementation of information systems to support a continuum of care is a new experience for Partners and the industry. It appears that the industry is still in the early stages of thought and experience gathering in both the formulation and implementation aspects of strategy development. Very fundamental questions and concepts remain to be resolved or clarified.

Knowledge of the high-leverage care improvement opportunities in continuum-based care processes remains limited. Preliminary data, presented earlier in this section, suggest that there are many leverage points and much leverage is needed. However, for example, the incidence, severity, and sources of outpatient medication errors are not well understood. Data regarding the utility of handheld outpatient medication prescription applications are limited. The ability of clinical information systems to improve the clinical component of the referral process lacks thorough analysis. The industry has insufficient understanding of how to deliver affordable clinical information systems to the small practice. Systems to support the capture of data for clinical trials and clinical research, while not unduly interfering with practice workflow, remain to be developed.

The value of integrated care is poorly defined. Integrated care would seem to promise fewer problems associated with incomplete information about the patient, more appropriate placement of the patient in care settings, and improved sharing of knowledge with providers. However, the value, in terms of both economics and care quality, of integrated care has not been well established.

Summary: Clinical Information System Concepts and Views

Provider order entry implementation provides an example of strategy formulation (the need to reduce medication errors as a focus of efforts to improve care) and implementation (the discussion of a series of IT asset changes.)

Improving the efficiency and effectiveness of care was (and still is) a strategic imperative of Partners. The IT response, derived from this linkage, largely focused on improving core organizational processes, centering, for the purpose of reducing ADEs, on the process of ordering. This order entry project also leveraged critical organizational data: the retrospective review of ordering patterns and the presentation of data to the ordering physician in a just-in-time fashion.

A series of strategies regarding the clinical information system applications asset emerged:

• Applications should focus on improving care processes that have been thoroughly studied, leading to a clear linkage between the care improvement opportunity and required IT capabilities.

• Care improvement is fated to be an ongoing, iterative set of analyses and interventions because our knowledge of what works and what doesn't work in care can be limited and our understanding of the impact of clinical systems on care improvement is often deficient. Internal development was deemed necessary to provide application agility.

Changes were made to the IT asset components of infrastructure, governance, IT staff, and data as well as the applications.

We also introduced the notion of "strategic views." These views are ideas and concepts that guide how we think about a strategy and the initiatives designed to effect it. In developing the BWH overall strategic response to the pressures on care delivery, two major organizational concepts were defined that form the core view of care: care as a process and the clinical management of care. These views generated three IT goals: improve care-centric processes, enhance patient and provider decision making, and measure the process of care.

The IT goals led to a core view or concept that guided the development of BWH and PHS clinical systems, in particular the provider order entry system: the information-rich process. While engaged in a process, such as a medication order, the IT application would deliver information needed to make appropriate decisions.

The design and implementation challenge confronted several sources of significant complexity that defy quick solutions. Each application endeavor must bound the complexity factors—for example, by focusing on standards for some but not all data and confining an application to an inpatient process.

Integration of Information Systems

As discussed in Chapter Three, the IT asset has characteristics. The governance structure can be decentralized or centralized. Data can be accurate or not. Organizations will always find that there are aspects of the asset that need to be improved or changed and hence will embark on activities designed to strengthen the asset.

Often the needed activities are straightforward to state, even if they are hard to implement. The IDS may decide to improve the consistency of its measures of care quality by tightening up the definitions of data. The organization may decide to improve the supportability of its infrastructure by investing in new, powerful network management tools.

There are other times when the asset characteristic is quite complex and difficult to define with precision and yet the characteristic is regarded as critical. In these cases, the organization would be well served if it spent time forming a thoughtful view of the definition and nature of the characteristic before it embarks on the commitment of resources directed to its "improvement." For example, agility would seem, at face value, to be a very important characteristic of applications and infrastructure (and the organization as a whole), but what does it really mean? What does agility look like? How much does agility cost? How would we assign a value to agility?

As organizations think strategically about and develop plans for their IT assets, several questions should be posed.

- What asset characteristics are important to us? Organizations often find all of the asset characteristics to be important to at least some degree. However, some characteristics are more important than others. This ranking of importance can be a reflection of today's issues and priorities. The integration of the infrastructure may be a more immediate concern than the agility of the infrastructure early in the life of an IDS. The ranking can also reflect a "normative" sequence of importance. If the data are highly inaccurate, the characteristics of accessibility and understandability may diminish to irrelevancy until the accuracy is made at least barely acceptable. The importance of asset characteristics can reflect the nature of the industry and its basis of competition. When the bases of competition varies by metropolitan area, a national health care provider may choose a governance structure that emphasizes local responsiveness.

- Can we define the characteristic crisply, or does the definition seem to be complex, multifaceted, and elusive? What does potency mean to us? What does data understandability mean? Assigning a definition (and a measure) to potency can be very difficult. Object technology would appear to be potent because it supports reusability of standard programs. But how would one know if one object offering was more potent than another? A definition of a common definition (understandability) of a data element, for example, primary care provider, would seem to be easy to develop. It is. But effecting it can be elusive because there are strong reasons that various constituencies have for their specific, crisp, and individually correct but collectively inconsistent definitions.

- If the definition is elusive or complex, what principles, views, and strategies should guide our pursuit of improving the characteristic? We may find it hard to define potency or to measure it. Nevertheless, we can decide to replace our technical infrastructure every four years because we believe that doing so will enable us to keep up with the most potent technology. We may not be sure how to define or measure an "innovative" IT organization, but we will undertake some of the steps outlined in Chapter Three.

- What is our plan for ensuring that the asset has the characteristics desired? What plans, tactics, and resources do we need to have in order to advance the asset? Is the plan straightforward or something less than that?

In the remainder of this section, we pursue the aspect of integration in the IT asset. Drawing from the experiences of Partners, we will cover two major aspects of integration:

- The application and infrastructure foundation for clinical integration across a delivery system
- Technical architecture integration strategies

Integration is an example of an asset characteristic for which the definition is complex, multifaceted, and elusive. Yet arriving at an integration strategy is crucial.

Integrated delivery systems are investing enormous energy and resources attempting to operationalize the word *integrated*. Although the industry is now full of "integrated delivery systems" developing "integrated care," it is not clear that we have a well-developed understanding of what that means. We have semi-fantastic descriptions of how it all might work, using lots of nifty words like *seamless* and *transparent*. But we lack a large number of real, pragmatic examples of continuum-based care really working at scale.

The value of integration is not well understood and is at times directly challenged (Herzlinger, 1997). An organization needs to create a technical and application infrastructure that allows it to adapt to integration as the organization develops a clear understanding of integration. Strategies that presuppose an understanding of integration, such as all participants using the same system, may be quite wrong. Understanding the meaning and value of integration will be an area of experimentation requiring application and infrastructure agility and organizational focus on measuring and evaluating experiences.

The IT integration effort is generally and correctly believed to require IDS efforts to integrate clinical, administrative, and financial information systems and system utilities such as electronic mail. A critical undertaking for the IT group of any IDS is to develop strategies for facilitating integration. Ideally, these strategies and tactics are effective, efficient, and capable of a high degree of leverage—for example, an interface engine that can be applied across a wide range of integration tasks.

Principles and Views That Guide Integration

The integration strategy at Partners is guided by six major concepts. These concepts form the cornerstones of its strategic view of integration.

- Constellations
- Transcendent core

- Focus on processes and data
- Integration as an idiosyncratic evolution
- Opportunistic movement
- Minimally invasive delivery of chunks

Constellations. Not all parts of an IDS need to be integrated with every other part. The physician practices surrounding a hospital may need to be well integrated with each other and with that hospital (collectively forming a constellation) but have less need to be integrated with another of the system's hospitals twenty miles away (forming another constellation). An IDS may have half a dozen constellations, each perhaps centered on an IDS hospital, distributed over a relatively large geographical area. There may be a lesser need to integrate between constellations than within a constellation.

For example, if 99 percent of the physician-to-physician referrals occur within a constellation, that process, and the related information systems, should be tightly integrated. If 1 percent of the referrals cross constellation boundaries, application integration across constellations need not be so tight; the referral can be faxed.

An IDS should focus on ensuring a high degree of integration within a constellation even if that means, for example, using a different vendor from the one chosen by another constellation. In Partners, for example, the North Shore Medical Center constellation uses one primary vendor, the Newton-Wellesley Hospital constellation uses another, and the Brigham and Women's constellation uses internally developed applications. In each case, the central focus is integration within a constellation. For Partners, since cross-constellation integration needs are modest, there is no compelling rationale for a common system across all constellations.

Transcendent Core. The degree of integration across constellations may be modest, and the central locus of integration may be the constellation. However, it may be clear, from the IDS strategy, that cross-constellation integration can be expected to increase, although the future forms of integration may not be well understood. Despite limited understanding, some integration applications may be obvious since the IDS cannot imagine a future where these applications would be irrelevant. For example, communication needs may demand a common telephone directory and a common e-mail system. Several visions of a continuum of care may point to a clinical data repository (CDR). This set of obvious capabilities is referred to as the "transcendent core" and has several properties:

- Each component of the core should be applicable across a wide range of future integration scenarios.

- The need for each component should be readily apparent, since funding may otherwise be difficult because of the fuzzy value of integration.
- In the early stages of the life of an IDS, the implementation of the core should not unduly interfere with efforts to improve constellation integration.

The Partners' transcendent core is described later in this chapter.

Focus on Processes and Data. To determine whether an integration need requires a common system, one should try to understand what processes and data form the basis of integration and whether there are degrees of integration. For example, IDS-wide financial reporting may require common definitions of certain pieces of data but perhaps not require common closing schedules or a common general ledger. Standardized care of asthmatics may require common protocols and measures of outcomes, but these can be implemented in systems offered by different vendors. The need for a composite clinical view of the care delivered across the system may require one IDS-wide clinical data repository and standards for its content but not require that hospital patient care systems be replaced.

By defining an IDS on the basis of the set of processes and data that link organizations, one also realizes that the organizational boundaries of an IDS are elusive; it is often not clear where the IDS "ends." Process-based and data-based integration needs will exist with organizations on the other side of the IDS boundary.

Integration as an Idiosyncratic Evolution. Integration will evolve as organizations understand where integration makes sense and where it doesn't. Organizations may integrate functions that will need to be disassociated later. They may establish some level of integration between functions and then change that level as they learn more. Organizations will go through several iterations, experiments, successes, and failures until they settle on a mature understanding of integration. This may take decades to accomplish.

The IDS IT organization will learn that integration can have many meanings, for example:

- A single password and look and feel for all systems
- The ability to access all IDS applications from any workstation in the IDS
- An interface between applications
- Common data definitions and a common database
- Common clinical and operational application processes, for example, a single way to determine eligibility across all entities in the IDS
- A single application system to support consolidated administrative functions

- Different implementations of the same application
- A single application to support the consolidation of a subset of ancillary departments, such as two out of four radiology departments
- A common application to support the integration of some clinical services but not others
- Various combinations of these things

There will be no one way to integrate systems. The nature of the integration needed will range from system access to a very tight coupling of applications. The IT organization will need to develop a set of integration tools and know which ones to apply in a multiplicity of situations.

A "single system" for all systems in an IDS may be prohibitive politically, economically, and temporally. It is not clear that a single system can accommodate the variation just described or that a single system improves the situation. A single system may require a degree of control over an affiliate's IT decisions that cannot be achieved. Similarly, an interface engine will be useful in some situations but not others. Common vocabularies for data will make sense in some situations—for example, the definition of a primary care provider—but create unnecessary work in others, such as reasons for visit no-shows.

At times one defines a phenomenon based on the tools that one has to address it. The presence of a diverse set of tools that are useful in certain contexts but not others means that the phenomenon is diverse and difficult to pin down. Such is the case with integration.

Opportunistical Movement. Often members of an IDS voice slogans—"Integration is good," "We want integrated systems"—without knowing what an integrated application should really do or how much money or effort is reasonable to expend in order to get one. One should be hesitant to integrate until it is clear what integration really means to the proponent and why it will be worth the trouble.

Integration may take time to emerge, but organizations should ensure that application, technology, and data decisions seize opportunities to ease (often future) integration needs. When selecting a new application, one should choose one from a vendor already installed at an IDS site. Organizations can demand that new applications conform to certain standards that ease integration.

The IDS can adopt a strategy of progressive or opportunistic homogeneity and integration. This strategy seeks out and capitalizes on opportunities to standardize processes, data, and technology or reduce organizational IT asset heterogeneity. Several examples exist:

- IDS concern with losing money on its medication risk arrangement provides an opportunity to standardize formularies and medication dictionaries.

- An organization in the IDS that wants to replace its radiology system provides an opportunity to choose a replacement system used by other organizations in the IDS.
- HIPAA regulations concerning a national provider identifier provide an opportunity to standardize that data element across the IDS.
- IDS concern with its management of hypertensive males provides an opportunity to rationalize that care process.

Progressive or opportunistic homogeneity does mean that integration may be somewhat idiosyncratic. However, it also means that organizational interest in achieving at least partial integration will be high.

Minimally Invasive Delivery of Chunks. When the process to be integrated spans constellations (or IDS boundaries), browser-based applications will often be used, and these may require, at most, only modest degrees of integration with existing constellation-based applications. This "minimally invasive" application delivery strategy can reduce the cost and accelerate the pace at which these integration applications can be delivered in various ways:

- By reducing the need to replace existing infrastructure (networks and workstations, for example) before extending an "integrating" application or process out to IDS member organizations. The expense of replacing infrastructure (and the time required) can thwart efforts to integrate.
- By layering a common process on top of an individual member organization's applications. This process may not be integrated at all with extant applications, thereby reducing the overhead of application interfacing or replacement. For example, the IDS may provide a common way to determine eligibility or request a referral. This noninterface approach can result in some degree of operational inefficiency that may be acceptable when cross-constellation integration is modest.

The IDS may also develop applications so that parts or "chunks" of the application can be delivered to a setting and not require that the full application be implemented. For example, some physicians' offices would benefit from the ability to edit a transcribed note but not need the fully computerized record, or a site may be interested in medication order entry but not procedure order entry. By allowing chunks to be implemented, an IDS may speed up delivery of information systems value, find a more receptive customer, and reduce the cost and complexity of integration. If the basis of process integration is 20 percent of an application, requiring the implementation of 100 percent can slow progress.

Clinical Integration at Partners

IT support has been necessary to effect a wide range of integrations undertaken at Partners HealthCare. Consolidation of the departments of Finance, Materials Management, and Human Resources led to a common PeopleSoft application across Partners entities. Fundamental needs to communicate and share files has led to a common electronic mail system (Outlook) and shared file areas.

We shall now discuss the integration of patient care, research, and education— or in Partners terminology, *clinical integration*. In developing its strategic plans, Partners identified eleven clinical integration goals, listed in Exhibit 4.1. Accountability for these goals was established, and teams and committees were formed to develop action plans for each goal.

Implementation of the information systems to support these goals proceeded through three stages:

- Definition of critical characteristics and capabilities
- Determination of the IT applications and infrastructure
- Development and execution of implementation plans

The first two stages are discussed together because they are not serial but run in parallel and interact with each other. Both stages focused on the transcendent core.

Critical Characteristics and Capabilities of Needed Information Systems. Information systems that support clinical integration need to do all of the following:

- Support a patient's care as the individual moves through the system by ensuring the accessibility of patient data throughout the Partners organization

EXHIBIT 4.1. CLINICAL INTEGRATION GOALS FOR PARTNERS HEALTHCARE SYSTEMS, INC.

- Develop a systemwide quality improvement agenda
- Oversee and facilitate implementation of Principles of Patient Flow
- Develop IS strategy to support clinical collaboration across the system
- Deploy PCHInet to PCHI physicians
- Connect nonacute care to the rest of the care continuum
- Develop strategy for integrating training between academic programs and between academic and community settings
- Deploy clinical trials systemwide
- Increase research collaboration among all Partners institutions
- Establish business plans for selected systemwide service lines
- Develop strategy for relationships with community specialists
- Develop a plan to align incentives for institutions, physicians, and administrators

- Support the "roaming" provider who might practice in several locations at Partners and who must be able to access his or her systems regardless of location
- Enable communication to take place among providers, patients, and other stakeholders
- Extend clinical applications and resources to specific communities, for example, a set of applications tailored to oncologists
- Streamline interorganizational care processes, for example, referrals or procedure-ordering processes
- Capture and promulgate knowledge and best practices on a wide range of care practices
- Enable quality to be measured and practice patterns and characteristics to be identified
- Support clinical research through, for example, the publication of information on clinical trials and the creation of databases to identify cohorts of Partners patients eligible for a trial
- Accommodate complex, idiosyncratic, and evolving service and care configurations; for example, the integration that occurs between any two Partners hospitals will be different, and evolve differently, from the integration between any other two hospitals
- Minimize the need to replace existing systems that work
- Minimize the demands for expensive infrastructure
- Provide high reliability, performance, supportability, confidentiality, and security of applications and infrastructure

These capabilities and characteristics guide infrastructure and application architecture and implementation decisions. For example, the need to minimize expensive infrastructure points to browser-based applications and virtual private network (VPN) technologies. Support for the roaming provider points to the need for a common security system. The ability to deliver care to a patient as he or she moves through the system requires that a computerized medical record exist to capture outpatient data.

Critical IT Components to Support Clinical Integration. A set of information systems applications and infrastructure, derived from the characteristics just described, became the foundation (the transcendent core) for clinical integration. These applications could support multiple integration efforts. For example, a common network infrastructure can be leveraged by multiple integration efforts. A common phone directory provides broad support for communication. Specific integrations such as the merger of two hospitals would have additional, specialized needs, but these specifics were not included in the definition of foundation. Moreover, several initiatives should leverage constellation initiatives, for example, support a constellation's need for a computerized medical record.

Implementation of the transcendent core began shortly after the Partners was formed and is likely to continue for the foreseeable future. The core has a dozen components.

• Universal access to applications and resources involves the development of a Partners workstation that supports access to a set of applications and services tailored to the role and privileges of the user. A Windows 95, Windows 2000, and Web version of the workstation have been developed. Workstation design included the implementation of a common security system. At this time there are 19,000 Partners workstations deployed and 37,000 devices (including nonstandard workstations) on the Partners network.

Universal access also involves the implementation of a common network. The reach of access has recently been extended by the development of a VPN to augment the scope of the core network that links the various Partners sites. In addition to networks and workstations, a common shared file area has been established. Figure 4.4 presents a diagram of the Partners network infrastructure.

FIGURE 4.4. PARTNERS NETWORK INFRASTRUCTURE.

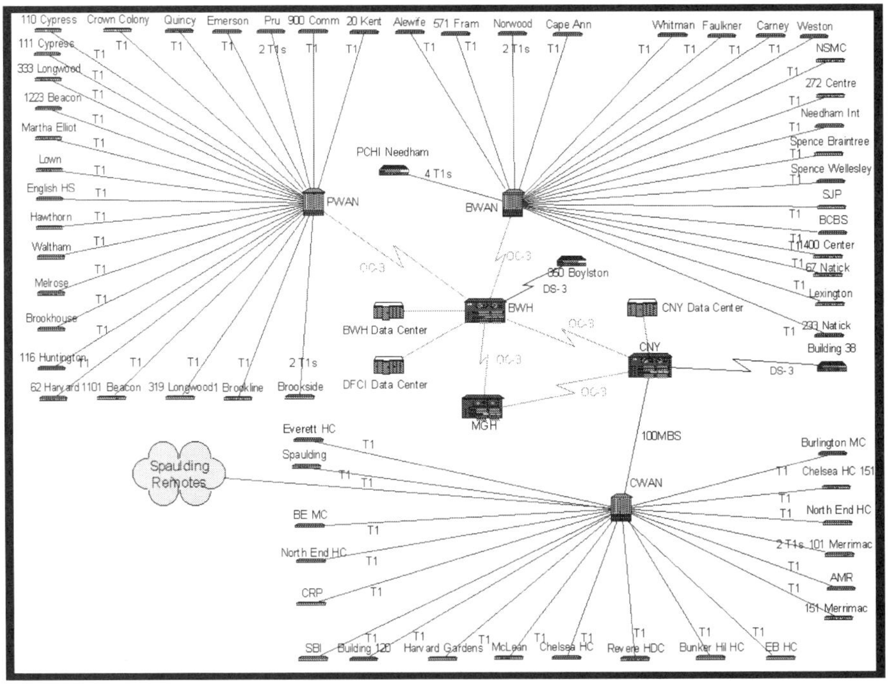

• Common Provider Master (CPM) provides a unique identifier for all Partners providers; it includes information such as practice location, specialty, and license numbers. Unique identification of providers helps in analysis of care practices, administrative activities, and the management of system privileges.

• Common communications provide core e-mail services (currently 47,000 accounts), a phone directory with a link to the paging system, a directory of all Partners physicians, and bulletin board and chat session support.

• Knowledge resources include external and internal references, guidelines and protocols, and in the future, direct consultation with a specialist. Figure 4.5 contains a screen from Handbook, the central location of Partners clinical knowledge resources. In this figure, Handbook has been accessed through the community physician portal, PCHInet. Partners Community HealthCare Inc. (PCHI) is the subsidiary of Partners that manages the Partners network of primary care providers and community specialists.

• Enterprise Master Person Index (EMPI) identifies an individual patient by his or her BWH, MGH, and other medical records numbers and currently contains 2.5 million records.

FIGURE 4.5. KNOWLEDGE RESOURCES (HANDBOOK).

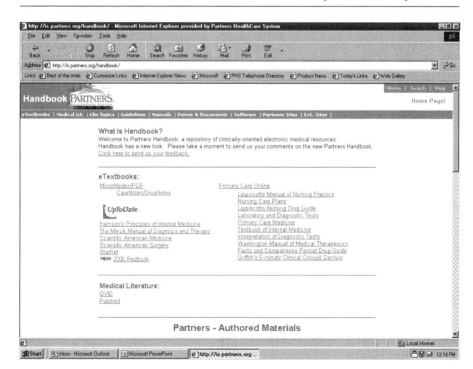

• The Clinical Data Repository (CDR) is an aggregate of all computer-based clinical data for patients with entries in the EMPI, downloaded from clinical information systems at Partners sites. The CDR currently contains, for example, 250 million test results and 7 million radiology reports. One hundred thousand results and reports are added to the repository daily. Figure 4.6 shows the viewer of CDR data.

• Enterprise Medical Imaging, or Picture Archival and Communication Systems (PACS), provides access to radiology and other images throughout the Partners organization. Approximately 40 million images are currently stored on-line. Figure 4.7 depicts the access of a medical image.

• The computerized ambulatory medical record (often referred to as the computerized patient record, or CPR), currently used by twelve hundred Partners physicians, improves operations and care in ambulatory settings. In addition to practice-specific value, the CPR supports integration in the following ways:

• Supporting capture of and access to a patient's outpatient clinical data as he or she moves through the system

FIGURE 4.6. CDR RESULTS VIEWER.

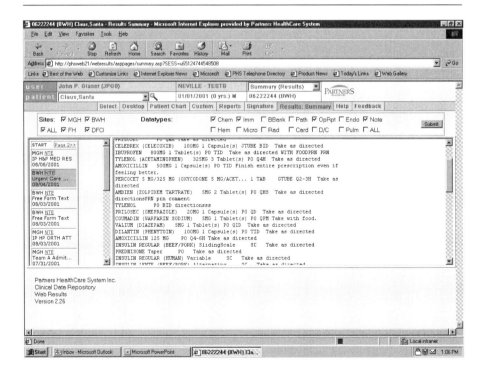

- Capturing data for quality measurement and research
- Supporting best care practices by reminding physicians to perform certain tests and complete documentation
- Structuring data collection to enhance the quality of care by guiding, for example, regular testing of certain parameters for patients with diabetes

Figure 4.8 shows the main screen of the CPR.

• "Community portals" use Web technologies to provide branded bundles of services and applications to a specific clinical community. Brands can include primary care physicians, Partners Mental Health, Brigham and Women's Hospital referring physicians, and Dana Farber/Partners Cancer Care (DF/PCC) oncologists. Some services, such as electronic mail, are common across all brands or communities, while other services, such as clinical trial registration for DF/PCC, are unique to a specific community. The computerized ambulatory medical record, medical imaging, and knowledge resources are other examples of applications and services that are delivered through such portals.

• The Research Patient Data Registry (RPDR) is formed through the extraction of data from the CDR, cost accounting, and other systems. The system can

FIGURE 4.7. VIEWING A MEDICAL IMAGE.

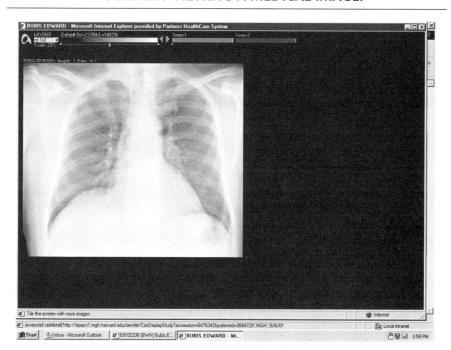

FIGURE 4.8. MAIN SCREEN OF THE COMPUTERIZED AMBULATORY MEDICAL RECORD.

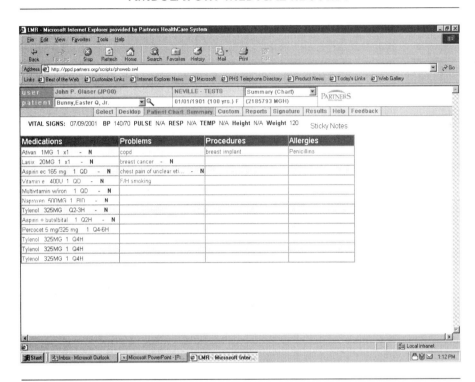

be queried by the clinical research community to identify candidates for clinical trials.

• Quality measurement and care analysis databases are used to assess care quality and identify variations in practice patterns; these include the University HealthSystem Consortium (UHC) Clinical Database and a data mart focused on cardiology care quality.

• Requests for interentity clinical services are care processes that span the boundaries of Partners organizations. Examples include referrals, procedure ordering, and requests for a patient transfer. These applications are Web-based and can be implemented with minimal integration with the information systems of the participating organizations. Figure 4.9 shows an example of application that enables a request for home health services.

Specific integrations require additional, individualized application support—for example, the merger of Union and Salem Hospitals, the integration of the

FIGURE 4.9. HOME HEALTH SERVICE REQUEST.

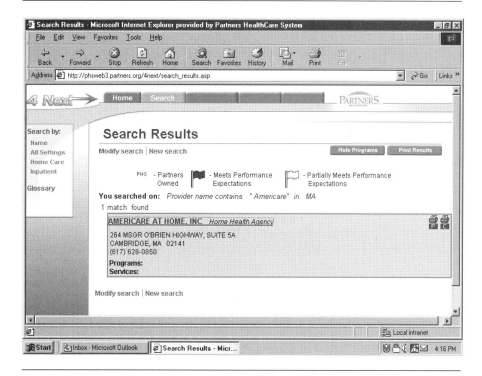

operating rooms of the Brigham and Faulkner Hospitals, and the creation of a network of nonacute care providers. Each of these subsets leverages the overall integration portfolio but has specific and unique purposes and integration needs.

Observations of IDS Clinical Integration. Applying information systems to further IDS integration is very difficult, complex, and nuanced. Early industry understanding of this challenge was limited and often naive. This is not to impugn the intelligence of the health care information systems community; rather it is a comment on how much there has been to learn.

IDS integration was initially described in the industry in terms of a single suite of applications, a single IT management structure, common processes, and well-defined organizational boundaries. However, Partners and other IDSes have become a confederation of organizations and a collection of idiosyncratic and opportunistic joint ventures, affiliations, and consolidations with poorly defined organizational boundaries. Information systems to support these complex organizations are vastly more complex than the systems needed by smaller, more homogeneous entities.

The health care information systems community has at times confused uniformity with integration. The implementation of the same pharmacy or laboratory or general ledger system across the IDS is neither always essential for integration nor inherently a furthering of integration. Nonetheless, when it needs to replace an application, an organization attempts to narrow the diversity of vendors, often by limiting the choice of vendors to those who already have a presence in the IDS. The narrowing of diversity should not lead the organization to believe that integration follows as an automatic outcome of diversity reduction.

IT integration strategies often place a premium on initiatives that preserve options in the future, in other words, initiatives that have value in a wide range of future IDS scenarios. It is hard to imagine an integration scenario under which sending an e-mail message to someone would be viewed as not an important contribution. Such initiatives must balance the cost and value of the initiative—for example, is it worth the "gamble" that this initiative will be deemed valuable in the future? The cost of the initiative must also consider the opportunity costs of investing in a still ill-defined integration initiative rather than redirecting the capital to specific, local hospital initiatives.

At the end of the day, information systems integrations should advance the strategies, goals, and performance of the IDS. However, while executing projects in the day-to-day mode, IT leadership needs to ensure that it is creating the broad ability to integrate more efficiently and effectively in the future. The IT organization will continue to need to respond to a diverse set of integration challenges. Organizational, management, and technical strategies and tactics need to be developed that can be efficiently and effectively applied to a range of challenges. Too often we focus on the projects that loom before us without sufficient management attention on the overall ability of the IT staff and the architecture to effect integration.

Technical Architecture Integration

The core concept guiding the Partners approach to the technical integration of the infrastructure and applications is the notion of levels. Levels reflect the observation that application and infrastructure integration needs can range from loosely coupled (being able to access an application) to tightly coupled (a common enterprisewide registration system). Our foregoing discussion of the clinical integration strategy provides examples of levels. Universal access is a loosely coupled approach to integration. The implementation of a common computerized medical record reflects a more tightly coupled level.

There are four levels, which reflect the discussion in Chapter Three on infrastructure capabilities:

1. The ability for a person to access, from anywhere within the IDS, his or her own applications and services, subject to user authorization. These applications and services may not be integrated with each other.
2. The ability to have a consistently defined set of data across the IDS. These data can be used for reporting purposes or as the basis of data exchange between two applications.
3. The ability to establish common processes across the IDS. A common process can be a referral, the identification of a patient, or the sending of an e-mail message with attachments.
4. The ability of applications to behave the same way across an IDS—for example, a common look and feel and command set or the implementation of the same application across all IDS organizations.

Several observations are important:

- As one goes from the first to the fourth level of integration, the degree of integration generally increases.
- Addressing one level invariably requires that one address at least some elements of the preceding levels.
- Work performed to address one level eases the work required to effect subsequent levels.
- The IDS can also adopt one level of integration for a class of systems or a portion of the IDS and another level of integration for another class of systems or different portion of the IDS. For example, two IDS members may have the same radiology system but across all four radiology departments the vocabulary of procedures may be standardized.
- Strategies carried out to support integration often support the improvement of other infrastructure characteristics; for example, standardizing the workstation and its operating system also enhances supportability.

Let us look at some strategies used at each of these levels.

Access Strategies. Access strategies generally require the development or identification of a number of things:

- A common presentation technology, for example, a browser or an IDS-wide Visual Basic front end

- Consistent names and definitions for the applications and services presented
- A common security service that maintains information on authentication, such as passwords, and authorization—in other words, what services and applications employees can access

Data Commonality Strategies. There are several data commonality strategies.

- Define common syntax and semantics. Data commonality strategies center on arriving at a common syntax for the exchange of information between applications, such as HL7 and ANSI X.12, and a common semantic that defines data meaning and coding conventions, such as ICD-9 for patient problems and LOINC for laboratory test results.
- Adopt exchange technology standards that provide the technical environment for the exchange of messages, transactions, or specific elements of data. Such technology standards might include XML or CORBAMed.
- Develop competency in a range of interfacing technologies. Interfacing technologies are diverse and vary in elegance. An IDS should be able to implement an interface engine, perform a screen scrape or a file transfer, and perhaps scan documents and printouts into machine-readable form.
- Move toward component-based and message-based architectures. The use of well-defined application components that expose their capabilities or services to other applications through well-defined messages will over time enable a marked improvement in application process interoperability. An IDS may evolve to the point where applications that need the identity of a patient or member are able to use a standard message exchange mechanism regardless of which vendor supplies the code that does the identification.

Common Process Strategies. Common process strategies are diverse and complex. This should not imply that arriving at a common semantic for clinical data across the IDS is a trivial task. The concepts of constellations, transcendent core, process and data focus, and minimally invasive delivery of chunks represent common process strategies. In addition to these strategies, other strategies can be defined:

- Limit the list of acceptable applications to some small number that, in addition to reducing the cost of these applications and improving supportability, can enhance integration if the integration supplier is told that winning the business requires the presence of integration technologies in the application and if the implementation of a common systems is used as a catalyst for standardizing data and processes.

• Develop a vendor anchor-tenant approach. In this approach, the IDS defines one vendor as the core supplier of its applications (the anchor). All other application vendors must coexist or integrate (as tenants) with the applications provided by the anchor vendor.

• Develop a process architecture. Common processes form the basis of a high degree of integration in an IDS. These processes can be common across the enterprise or between some groups of IDS members. While it may not be clear how an IDS will achieve these common processes, it will have a better chance of arriving at "commonness" if it has a fairly clear definition or architecture of the processes and related subprocesses (Drazen and Metzger, 1998). This architecture requires that the processes be defined—for example, engage and retain members, assess health, and develop care and wellness plans. Moreover, the related subprocesses must be defined. Subprocesses of the "develop care and wellness plans" process might include set standards and monitor performance, develop a wellness plan, develop a care plan, and engage and manage referrals.

Reasonably detailed subprocess flow narratives and mock computer screens can be developed (Drazen and Metzger, 1998). This process architecture serves to guide specific implementation decisions.

Consistent Application Behavior Strategy. If the IDS desires that any of its staff can go to any of its sites and use the applications the same way that they would at any other site, a common system commonly implemented would be needed. The delivery of "chunks" would also help ensure that a process has consistent behavior across the enterprise.

Summary: Integration of Information Systems

We have examined integration examples of formulation and implementation. For clinical integration, formulation involved determination of critical characteristics and capabilities. For infrastructure integration, four levels of integration were developed. For clinical integration, implementation involved the definition of the elements that composed the transcendent core. For infrastructure integration, specific data and transaction standards were outlined.

The clinical integration IT agenda was developed to respond to a suite of organizational clinical integration strategies. The agenda focused on improving the broad asset property of integration of applications, infrastructure, and data in a manner that should provide utility under a range of future integration scenarios. The infrastructure IT agenda was similarly developed as a response to a broad organizational imperative to integrate and focused on improving the integrability of the infrastructure. The resulting levels create a kind of "integration tool kit."

The integration-centric efforts we discussed were centered on multiple components of the IT asset, emphasizing infrastructure and applications. However, several of the components of the transcendent core contributed to the improvement of the data asset, including the timeliness and accessibility of outpatient data that can result from the CPR. In addition, an IT department, Enterprise Services, was created to manage several aspects of clinical integration: EMPI, CDR, RPDR, quality measurement, and CPM. The department also monitors overall progress on the IT clinical integration agenda.

Finally, we saw the notion of views regarding integration. For clinical integration, views included concepts such as constellations, transcendent core, and minimally invasive delivery of chunks. The views also included the determination of critical capabilities and characteristics. For technical architecture integration, the concept of levels forms the dominant view. One can see that a different set of views might lead one to a very different IT response. For example, if the concept of constellations was deemed a bad idea, an IDS-wide single system might result. If an organization decided that only the first level was relevant, a common network and application access mechanism might be the extent of the IT response.

The Internet

From time to time, information technologies emerge that have the ability to significantly influence the strategies and plans of an organization or the manner in which the organization architects its infrastructure and applications. Examples of these technologies include transistors, time-sharing, networks, bar codes, global position satellites, and the personal computer. There is also the steady emergence of information technologies that, while important, have not had a widespread impact on organizations and their information systems; these include CASE technologies and artificial intelligence.

A critical component of strategy development for IT is to understand, for a given new technology, whether it belongs in the first cohort or the second and why. An organization that miscategorizes runs the risk of either investing heavily in a technology that is unable to provide a commensurate leverage of the organization or missing an opportunity to take advantage of a technology that can help effect significant organizational changes or improvements.

In analyzing new technologies, the organization needs to answer five primary questions:

1. What are the core capabilities of the new technology? This is a simple question to state. But the answer must demonstrate insight and be based on essen-

tial capabilities of the technology. For example, the core capabilities of an airplane can be stated as follows:

- It allows one to go from point A to point B in less time than other modes of transportation.
- It does not require that a track or a road be in place and hence it costs less to achieve scope (go to lots of places) and can achieve greater range (go to places where it is impractical to create tracks and roads, for example, the jungle).

The core capability of refrigerators is that they allow perishable goods to last longer before they spoil. The global position satellite enables one to know, with great precision, where something is located anywhere on the globe. The transistor enables us to miniaturize a computer, greatly reduce the cost of the machine, significantly improve a computer's reliability and design, and create more complex circuits.

The definition of core capabilities is critical if an organization is to begin to understand how the technology might contribute and if the contribution will be significant.

2. What roles or general categories of use does the technology appear to fill? In other words, given the core capabilities, how might the technology be applied in an organization? For example, bar codes can fill several roles:

- Track an object as it moves from place to place
- Identify an object so that it can be linked to other data—for example, the bar code on a can of soup can be linked to current price information
- Serve as a "permanent," nonmagnetic storage device that can be applied to irregularly shaped objects

Global position satellites would enable us to know where a truck or railroad car is located. This is important if we have lost track of the railroad car, as in the case of a railroad car of bananas left on a side track a thousand miles from its destination. This knowledge of location can also enable us to reroute—for example, request the driver of a truck that is on the outskirts of a town to stop and pick up a last-minute order.

The capabilities of client-server technology enabled it to fill variety of roles, including these:

- Allowing multiple applications and systems to "seamlessly" use scarce or expensive "services" such as fax, slide making, database management, and high-volume printer services

- Permitting an application to use extensive logic checks, which run on another computer (the server), of a transaction without slowing down the entry of the transaction on the client

Organizations should note that the distinction between roles and core capabilities can be blurry.

3. What futures and opportunities can these roles create? Would these futures reflect significant or fundamental changes in our world and our organization?

Improved efficiency in routing and rerouting trucks offers an enormous advantage in a price-competitive and service-intense business.

Air conditioning enabled the vacation business in the southeastern United States to flourish. Families from the Northeast could enjoy their vacation in greater comfort.

Television altered the way news was reported, affecting the conduct of the Vietnam and Persian Gulf Wars.

Time-sharing enabled many organizations to extend services to their customers. The result was a significant leap in the competitive position of the organizations.

Refrigeration enabled the modern supermarket to offer meat and produce from many regions and countries rather than only from local agriculture. Refrigeration enables the delivery of medicines and antibiotics around the globe, resulting in major advances in the treatment of disease.

4. What have early uses of this new technology by others taught us? If the organization is not the first adopter or an early adopter, it should ask about the experiences of others. Are there some types of uses that are more successful than others? What troubles or disappointments have been encountered? To what degree are the disappointments the result of inexperience, inferior implementations of the technology, or technology immaturity rather than flaws in the technology concepts? For example, early efforts to fly were plagued with crashes and pilots who got lost. Early client-server implementations were difficult to manage, expensive, and unreliable. These problems were a reflection of the immaturity of the technology rather than any lack of merit in the concepts themselves.

5. Given the foregoing, how should we, a health care organization, pursue the technology? How should we incorporate the technology into our strategies? In answering these questions, the organization develops a strategy for the application and implementation of the technology. The tone of the strategy can range from radical change in the organization, perhaps because the organization sees the technology as disruptive (Christensen, 1997), to ignoring the technology because the roles and futures enabled by the technology are seen as trivial. The form of the strategy can range from aggressive adoption to the initiation of pilots and prototype development.

The answers to these five questions can vary from industry to industry and organization to organization. Bar codes are strategically important to retailers and less important to a law office. Some payers have aggressively pursued the Internet, while others are more cautious.

The Internet is an example of a new information technology that might have significant strategic implications for a health care provider organization. There is evidence, before one even answers the five questions, that something powerful is occurring. According to a survey conducted by the Pew Internet and American Life Project (2000):

- 55 percent of all U.S. Internet users have gone on-line for health or medical information, more than have shopped on-line.
- Of those who sought health or medical information, 32 percent looked for such information at least once a week.
- Of those who sought health or medical information, 9 percent have communicated with a doctor on-line, and 10 percent have described a medical condition or problem in order to get advice from an on-line doctor.

In the discussion that follows, we pursue the answers generated by Partners to the five questions with respect to the Internet.

Core Technical Capabilities of the Internet

The Internet has four core technical capabilities that are significant:

- The Internet uses an existing nearly ubiquitous and open network. Internet access leverages, and goes beyond, the phone system network. The Internet is now moving to the airwaves. Moreover, little incremental capital is required for an individual consumer or a service provider to become part of that network.
- Internet-based systems are minimally invasive of the client, workstation, or personal digital assistant. Hence the provider of Internet-based services and information is not concerned with the cost of supporting remote hardware or network connections. Nor do suppliers of Internet services confront the need to homogenize the workstation base in order to effect widespread use of their services.
- The Internet uses a very standard environment, such as HTML or HTTP. Hence Internet developers are reasonably sure that their software will work on the Internet and have a sufficient level of interoperability with other Internet offerings.
- Adding a new service to the Internet is trivial. A URL created today can be found by millions of browsers tomorrow. This is both a strength (we can be on

the Internet tomorrow) and a weakness (hundreds of our competitors can be on the Internet tomorrow).

The Internet and Internet technologies are less remarkable for their sophistication as technology than they are for the possible impact of that technology on society. The ability to create a spark (and hence a fire), using flint, on demand and the movable type set are examples of technologies that had remarkable social ramifications far in excess of the sophistication of the technology.

Roles of the Internet

The Internet can play a major role in three classes of organizational activity: information distribution, service provision, and process extension. These activities have core characteristics that the Internet can, because of its technical capabilities, alter or leverage, at times significantly. By altering these characteristics, organizations can materially change how they perform these activities.

The distinction between the three activities can be fuzzy, and one often finds that a specific Internet application leverages all three.

The core characteristics of information distribution include currency, reach, potency, and the marginal cost of distributing information. The telegraph changed the currency of information, changing forever, among other things, the nature of newspapers, markets for precious metals such as gold, and the way countries fight wars. Information about an event, which used to take weeks or months to cross continents, could be transmitted in seconds (Standage, 1999). Radio altered the reach of entertainment and news; one could listen to a comedian while relaxing at home. Television expanded the potency of information, combining video with audio, leading to a richer information experience. The printing press reduced the marginal cost of producing information (it is cheaper to produce the next book using the printing press than having a person copy it by hand), leading ultimately to universities and the creation of the middle class (Drucker, 2000). The Internet can change information distribution along all four characteristics.

Service industries can find that their world has changed dramatically due to alteration of service reach, the efficiency of richness, finding strategies, and the consumer's definition of "basic service." Reach is a measure of the number of customers who can access the service; for example, hundreds of millions of people can access vacation-planning services via the Internet (Evans and Wurster, 2000). Efficiency of richness refers to the cost, to the service organization, of providing a service experience tailored to the customer. The Internet, for example, has enabled the partial replacement of the expensive stockbroker by a Web site. Patients can find health care services and providers through mechanisms other than the recommendation of their physician or neighbor. The Internet enables customers to obtain service twenty-four hours a day and from millions of locations, leading the customer to expect that all services operate this way.

Organizations can use the Internet to extend critical processes to important business partners. Process extension has long been a major use of IT, as evidenced by the SABRE and ASAP systems. Process extension is the centerpiece of efforts to use the Internet to streamline the supply chain, construct electronic markets, and provide health insurance electronic data interchange. The Internet facilitates process extension by creating a common technology platform, for example, HTTP and XML, among all partners. Moreover, when there are a very large number of partners, the ubiquity of the Internet makes it easier to achieve scale. Nonetheless, the Internet will not solve critical aspects of large-scale process extension, for example, a lack of transaction standards or the integration of a heterogeneous base of partner legacy systems.

Possible Internet Futures

Given the information distribution, service provision, and process extension roles of the Internet, one can imagine a range of futures in health care.

Group purchasing organizations may see their position threatened by Internet-based auctions and aggregators of purchasers' requests for proposals to meet their supply needs. For example, several hospitals interested in IV solutions may come together in cyberspace to execute a onetime, item-specific group purchase. Suppliers, interested in the business, would find that the group purchasing organization has been replaced by these self-forming groups (possibly aided by an intermediary such as Medpool.com). In addition, the Internet might streamline the electronic connections that exist between purchasers, suppliers, and distributors (difficult though this streamlining may be). Finally, the Internet makes it easier for purchasers and suppliers to find each other, reducing some of the expense faced by smaller suppliers of establishing purchaser awareness of their existence.

Managed care organizations may find new competitors in the form of insurance "infomediaries." These infomediaries can offer many of the insurance functions of enrollment, benefit management, and claims management without the need for a local, physical presence. These infomediaries could erode the role of the insurance broker by directly reaching the employer. Infomediaries may be able to outsource third-party administration functions, achieving high economies of scale. Managed care organizations will also face great pressure to improve service to employers and subscribers through the use of Internet-based offerings, for example, enrollment and benefits management services.

The empowered consumer, having gleaned health-related information from the Internet, may cause several significant changes in the world of the provider:

- Consumers may find chat sessions and Internet communities to be more accessible and supportive sources of information than their primary care providers. The providers' role as the trusted authority may be eroded.
- Consumers, being made aware of the credentials and capabilities of the academic medical center specialist, may bypass the gatekeeper (primary care provider) and local specialist and directly seek care by an "international authority." The neighbor's recommendation of a specialist may be replaced by the recommendation of a fellow patient made in the course of a chat session. This trend would be supported by managed care relaxation of constraints surrounding referrals.
- Consumers may engage in spot market purchases of certain procedures and tests. For example, a patient with an injured knee may believe that he or she needs an MRI and consequently search the Internet for a convenient and inexpensive source for the MRI.
- As consumers experience the availability of around-the-clock, location-irrelevant services, such as buying a book or planning a vacation, they may push providers to increase the level of customer service. If I can arrange a vacation from my home at 2 A.M., why can't I schedule a physical?

The Internet can enhance the ability of organizations to craft inter- and intra-organizational relationships. Provider organizations can assist their efforts to integrate care through the implementation of extranets that provide e-mail, knowledge resources, and access to patient data. The Internet could be used to support provider and payer efforts to streamline the processes that bind them—for example, insurance transactions such as eligibility determination and claim status inquiry—and establish processes that they share—for example, a shared medical management function. The Internet can be used to craft new business relationships such as a provider and pharmacy benefits manager (PBM) cooperating to improve medication management by integrating provider order entry systems with PBM databases of patient medication claim history.

Clinical research could be enhanced by using the Internet to support clinical trial patient accruals and the sharing of data and clinical trials management software between organizations engaged in multisite clinical trials.

Physician compensation may change if patient encounters via e-mail and remote consultations grow significantly. Electronic encounters may reduce the number of physical encounters and enable the provider to carry a larger patient panel.

Specialists may find an erosion in geographical boundaries as they conduct second opinions over the Internet.

These futures may not all occur. Significant barriers and challenges confront the realization of many of them, and it is not clear that these futures are desirable. Nonetheless, they are all credible futures. An indication of the potency of any new technology is the range of credible futures. Technologies whose impact can be predicted with great certainty are inherently less potent than those that enable a wide range of futures.

History has shown us that it is difficult to predict the future that results from the implementation of profound technologies. The second- and third-order effects of profound technologies such as the automobile, the internal combustion engine, and flight were hard to imagine accurately when each technology was first introduced. In the early 1900s, few people understood that the automobile would lead to suburbs, an emptying of the inner city, the modern vacation industry, drive-in movie theaters, and shopping malls (Malone and Rockart, 1991). Similarly, the full impact of the Internet on health care is difficult to see with great clarity. How will the empowered consumer change health care delivery?

Flight exemplifies the mix of optimism and pessimism that confounds the futures discussion of profound technologies early in their lives. Many a science-fiction writer in the early twentieth century thought that our cities would someday have "air taxis" cruising several hundred feet in the air. Others, watching pilots get lost or planes crashing with great regularity, thought that the airplane would go nowhere.

Learning from Others

We now have several years of Internet experience across a range of industries to draw on. The experiences have included notable successes, such as achieved by Cisco and Dell (Dell, 1999). A large number of books and articles have been written to guide organizations in their application of the Internet (for example, Tapscott, 1998). And perhaps more numerous than the successes, the experiences have included notable failures—witness the demise of hundreds of dot-coms and the difficulties encountered in several industries with the construction of market exchanges ("Internet Pioneers," 2000).

These experiences have provided several broad lessons:

• The impact of the Internet has varied by industry and companies within industries. The music distribution, financial services, and retail industries have seen more of an Internet impact than organized religion, the legal profession, and the restaurant industry. Retailers of books have seen more of an impact than retailers of jewelry.

• Knowledge of how to apply the Internet and leverage the strategies of an organization is still very immature. Many assumptions about the impact of the Internet have been revealed as naive. It is difficult to disintermediate individuals and organizations that actually provide value. It can be very hard to connect thousands of suppliers to thousands of buyers. The economic savings of not having to deliver a paper newspaper can be overwhelmed by the IT costs of maintaining a news Web site. There is still significant room for experimentation and learning.

• The Internet efforts that have been successful have focused on the core sources of IT advantage discussed in Chapter Two: leveraging processes, obtaining critical organizational data, and product and service differentiation and creation.

- Amazon.com has arguably revolutionized the retail industry by making the process of buying a book more convenient. Moreover, Amazon uses data about prior purchases to suggest books (and other merchandise). Amazon enables book readers to leave their critiques of books for other readers, providing a differentiation of the book purchasing experience.
- Internet-based markets and exchanges intend to reduce the cost of goods and the cost of the purchase process. The markets should also make it easier for buyers and sellers to find each other.
- Internet-based procurement of office supplies makes that process more convenient and enables organizations to exert more control over the process.
- Distance learning is often directed to improving the convenience and accessibility of mid-career education. The educational offering could be tailored to the pace, mobility, and learning style of the student, differentiating the education. Many graduate programs are experimenting with this use.
- Contests lead teenagers (and maybe some adults) to Web sites to see if the number under a beverage cap has won a prize. At the Web site, valuable data about the beverage consumer is captured.
- Travel reservation Web sites are intended to ease the process of arranging travel or a vacation. Having the consumer conduct the transaction reduces the cost to the airline or hotel. Data entered by the traveler enable the site to be tailored to the individual and provides valuable information to the service provider.

• The boundaries between "Internet-based" applications and "regular" applications have become blurred. Internet applications often extend regular applications, and regular applications are often critical to effective Internet applications. For example, a Web site to order children's toys needs a regular materials management application to handle toy inventory and logistics. The use of a Web-based application to provide access to clinical data to a referring physician needs a hospital information system to serve the data. Rarely does one find a "pure" Web-based application that has no need for a "regular" application in order to be effective. And one finds that most, but not all, regular applications can be made more potent by extending them through Web technologies.

• The effectiveness of Internet applications is highly dependent on the thoughtfulness of an organization's strategy and the intelligence of its approach to leveraging core activities. For a while, the Internet jargon of "the New Economy," "Internet time," "business to business," and "business to consumer" implied that traditional management thinking and strategy prowess were irrelevant. A new way of thinking was necessary if one was going to thrive in cyberspace. But profits, knowing your customer, thinking long and hard about how to improve a process, and skillful organizational change and execution matter as much in the new economy as they do in the old economy (Porter, 2001). All of the ideas in this book of linkage and IT asset are just as important for an Internet-based application as they were for the time-sharing-based application of American Airlines. This observation also implies that a separate Internet strategy discussion is as problematic as a "regular" IT strategy discussion that has been separated from the normal management strategy discussion.

• Finally, the lessons illustrate the diversity of applications of the Internet. Perhaps this is not surprising since there are very diverse industries, organizations, and activities involved in information distribution, service delivery, and process extension. A health care organization will find a very wide range of possible Internet opportunities, some more potent than others, but a wide range nonetheless.

A view of the Internet emerges from the discussion up to this point:

• The Internet has a small number of powerful technical capabilities.
• The Internet may have a profound effect on health care organizations and core delivery because of its potential roles in information distribution, service delivery, and service extension. This effect will be more evolutionary than revolutionary because of the complex social, regulatory, and reimbursement environment of health care, which dampens the rapid adoption of many technologies.
• One can imagine futures that leverage these capabilities and roles that are very different from the world today. However, these futures are inherently uncertain, and achieving several of them is likely to be very difficult. Several of these futures will not materialize.
• Pursuing this powerful but fuzzy and risky future will require a thoughtful but bold, prudent but risk-tolerant, multifaceted strategy. This strategy should focus on those areas of organizational information distribution, service delivery,

and process extension where significant advances in reach and efficiency of richness matter.

Management Pursuit of an "Internet Strategy"

Health care delivery systems can begin to develop an "Internet strategy" by establishing organizational visions of an Internet future. This vision should be inclusive of non-Internet aspects of information technology, recognizing the Internet-regular application leverage.

Visions of the future are important; they serve as guides. Visions guide, and are molded by, necessary experimentation and learning. Organizational agility becomes essential as organizations must frequently fine-tune their course, progressively discovering and shaping the second-order and third-order world in which they will live.

Profound technologies and murky futures pose significant challenges as management attempts to establish strategies, create plans, and expend capital thoughtfully. Often this challenge is framed as a blanket statement: "We need an Internet strategy!" Perhaps a more effective statement is "We need to examine our strategy and our future in the context of our vision of what the Internet might mean."

This exercise of developing an Internet future and of crafting an Internet strategy should also recognize that this is a transient planning undertaking. In other words, once a reasonable vision and plans have been established, Internet strategy development should cease as a separate planning process. That vision should be folded back into the normal strategy development process. Separating a technology strategy conversation from a normal strategy conversation can be worthwhile when the technology is poorly understood by the organization. The separation enables the organization to focus on the new technology and develop its understanding of the technology's potential. However, once developed, the separation should end, or one risks an IT-strategy misalignment. Years ago, organizations often formed separate personal computer committees and personal computer planning processes. They needed to do this in order to develop an understanding of what was then a new and poorly understood technology. However, personal computer committees no longer exist, reflecting the fact that organizations have developed a sufficient understanding of personal computers to fold them back into the normal IT and organizational conversation.

To create the needed vision and guide the organization's use of the Internet, strategy questions should include the following:

• Does the Internet—and more specifically, use of the Internet—cause some of the fundamental assumptions that lie behind what we do to be no longer true?

For example, we may regard our competitors as our local colleagues and rivals. The Internet may expand the pool of potential competitors by including those who are located far away. We may find that Internet-based chronic disease communities become a trusted authority that weakens our physicians' role as that authority.

• Could we apply the Internet to materially improve our ability to carry out our current strategies? For example, can the Web enable us to be vastly more effective in our strategy to increase referrals from community physicians? Can we apply the Internet to improve the performance of our disease management programs?

• Can we significantly improve core activities and processes? Can Internet-based supply exchanges reduce the cost of purchasing supplies? Can the Web improve our ability to reduce medication errors in the ambulatory setting?

• What are others doing in our industry? What are our competitors doing? Do they have ideas and initiatives that we can learn from and make our own?

As is always the case, strategy questions must strike a delicate balance between keeping an open mind to new ideas that may identify current wisdom that is no longer wise and warranted cynicism toward intellectually flabby slogans.

In reviewing assumptions, strategies, and core processes, organizations will find Internet-based opportunities that appear to have great power. At times the power will favor the organization; for example, the Web can advance the integration of care across settings. At times the power may not favor the organization, as when "empowered" patients bypass their primary care provider and directly seek the advice of a specialist or a competitor they have found on the Web. Porter (2001), using the competitive forces model reviewed in Chapter Two (refer to Figure 2.5), notes that the Internet generally has negative effects on the five forces. In other words, the Internet will make most industries more competitive.

Organizations should be prudent in their choice of paths that arise from an Internet strategy conversation. Prudence would mean all of the following:

• Experimenting with new ideas to ensure that the opportunities, infrastructure to support them, and value to the organization are understood. Several e-tailers failed to understand order fulfillment and have suffered.

• Preparing the organization for change and managing that change. The same skill required to prepare an organization for life under managed care or for care based on clinical pathways is required for a substantive Internet-based change.

• Leveraging existing information systems, organizational processes, and people. Many organizations learned, through harsh lessons, the difficulty of radical change that began with a "clean organizational slate." Few organizations are actually clean slates; good people, who are good at what they do, occupy them ("The 2001 HBR List," 2001).

• Remembering that the Internet is still quite technically crude and currently ill equipped to support complex, mission-critical applications (National Research Council, 2000). Most Internet applications are in their infancy, and application maturity will take time to arrive.

• Remembering that while health care provider organizations should aggressively pursue their strategic examination of the Internet, the impact of the Internet is likely to be more evolutionary than revolutionary in health care. Nonetheless, fossils illustrate that evolution has resulted in victims.

So far, we have highlighted the possible role of the Internet in leveraging information distribution, service, and process extension. We have established that the Internet should be subject to the same management questions of impact on strategy and core processes that would be asked of any major innovation. In addition, an Internet strategy must bear in mind the observations presented here on the need for experimentation, managing change, and leveraging existing assets. The management response is neither radical nor passive. The form of the response will be a combination of pilots, to garner organizational experience and knowledge, and full resource commitment where the path is clear.

The Partners Internet Strategy

The Internet strategy development process at Partners had four goals:

• To understand the market factors that might shape or lead to Internet-based change. The impact of the Internet will be moderated and accelerated by factors other than the technology—for example, growth in the number of chronically ill, extent of home use of personal computers, and employer efforts to introduce greater use of defined-contributions health insurance.

• To identify Internet opportunities, issues, and possible threats. Planners were particularly interested in determining areas where the Internet could be used to significantly leverage Partners strategies, plans, and core processes. If the opportunity was uncertain, what pilots should be undertaken to garner early knowledge of the opportunity? The Internet was also likely to introduce new issues, for example, ensuring that patient-provider use of e-mail was conducted in a fashion that improved care delivery rather than undermined it. Finally, Partners might be threatened by the Internet efforts of others; for example, patient-directed payer health information that conflicted with the information delivered by a Partners provider or a geographically distant specialist offering second opinions in eastern Massachusetts.

- To determine the strategies and plans necessary to capitalize on the Internet. Given a list of opportunities, the associated IT and organizational plans and resources had to be defined.
- To promote a broad, sustained organizational examination of the role of the Internet. Since the effects of potent technologies play out over long periods of time, there would have to be a mechanism for ensuring that Internet strategy development became a core, ongoing set of strategy and management activities.

Structure of the Planning Process. Because of the possibility that the Internet might hold out significant opportunities (and threats), the committee overseeing the development of the strategy was chaired by the Partners CEO and was made up of board members and medical and administrative leaders.

To arrive at a first strategy, several paths or vectors were pursued. In general, when confronted with a complex phenomenon that has a wide range of credible futures, an organization should pursue the development of a strategy from several different perspectives. A strategy conclusion is likely to be more robust if it is derived through different paths and starting points. The Internet strategy at Partners was pursued from the following directions:

- Examination of opportunities for specific functions—for example, materials management or management of the chronically ill
- Review of the ability to leverage the Internet to achieve specific Partners goals—in other words, Internet initiatives derived directly from the organization's strategic goals
- Discussions at each of the member organizations of Partners to identify their perspective of the ability of the Internet to help address challenges specific to them
- Brainstorming sessions during which multidisciplinary teams were asked to define a set of desirable and adverse futures
- Review of the strategies and business visions of health care dot-com organizations
- Review of the strategies and Internet plans of other health care organizations and a sample of non–health care organizations
- Discussions with consultants, review of the literature, and listening to the ideas of speakers at conferences

These analyses led to the identification of nine areas where the Internet might have a significant impact on Partners:

- Remote consultations and second opinions—specialists at Partners consulting to physicians across the globe and within the United States

- Patient-provider interaction, ranging from patient-provider e-mail to remote monitoring of the chronically ill
- Payer relationships—Internet-based electronic data interchange, payer-provider process improvement, and possible integration of payer and provider Web sites
- Marketing and patient channeling—using the Internet to extend brand and help patients find Partners physicians and services
- System integration—integration of the Partners delivery system (discussed earlier in this chapter)
- Internal administrative process improvement—using Web technologies to distribute information and knowledge and to reduce the cost and improve the convenience of administrative transactions such as filing expense reports
- Supply chain and materials management—improving the ability to reduce the costs of supplies and integrating the Partners materials management processes with those of suppliers and distributors
- Research—pursuing opportunities ranging from the accrual of patients for clinical trials to the utilization of remote, scare equipment and resources such as electron microscopes
- Medical and health professional education—delivery of continuing medical education and distance learning for allied health degree candidates

To illustrate the nature of the Partners Internet plans, let's take a closer look at the plans for the first four areas.

Remote Consultations and Second Opinions. The Internet enables a physician to render a second opinion or remote consultation to a provider and patient anywhere on the globe. Some specialties, such radiology, oncology, neurosurgery, and cardiology, are more conducive to remote second opinions (where the physician need not see the patient) than others. Over time, these second opinions may account for 5 percent of the volume for those specialties.

Formidable barriers confront any effort to do this within the United States; these barriers include state licensure laws, lack of insurance coverage for this service, malpractice limitations, and the need for such a service to alter existing referral relationships in remote locales. Nonetheless, one should assume that those barriers will gradually be eliminated and Internet use for second opinions will become a standard practice.

Different barriers exist to offering second opinions internationally. Relationships need to be established with local organizations—for example, a government, managed care organization, or provider organization—that would initiate the referrals. These second opinions may lead to patients seeking care at Partners. Hence a Partners organizational unit must exist that can support such visits, for example, arranging for translator services and assisting patients with special dietary or religious needs.

The strategy concluded that despite the barriers, an organization such as Partners, which has a large base of specialists, will need to garner some experience with this form of Internet-based care. This experience should be in the form of limited but scalable pilots and investments.

The plan that resulted, for the United States market, can be summarized as follows:

- Conduct pilots in neurology, neurosurgery and oncology
- Provide "advertising" of this service on the Web sites of these departments (minimizing the marketing costs of the service)
- Require patient payment for the service (for which insurance coverage will not exist)
- Require that the patient engage his or her local physician in the second-opinion interaction (to address state licensure restrictions and to ensure that there is appropriate treatment follow-up)
- Develop the Web application needed to capture patient information and deliver the second opinion. (Figure 4.10 depicts a prototype, called eConsult, of a consulting physician's second opinion.)
- Create an internal second-opinion service department to manage this function

Patient-Provider Interaction. The Internet can be used to support and improve the interactions between patient and provider. There are three classes of patients, each class having different interaction needs: the well, the chronically ill, and the medically fragile.

The well patient has occasional needs to engage in transactions to request an appointment, refill a prescription, or ask a question. In addition, the patient will seek access to health information and have questions about insurance coverage. The physician's practice will need the ability to manage the incoming transactions and ensure that the patient knows how to use the offering. An Internet-based application can support these needs. Such an application should be fundamentally viewed as an opportunity to improve service.

The chronically ill patient, such as a person with epilepsy, will have the same needs as the well patient. In addition, such patients will seek access to information on clinical trials and new treatment options for their disease. They are likely to be interested in access to communities of fellow patients and to highly focused health information. They may also need access to certain types of commerce; for example, a stroke victim may be interested in housekeeping and shopping services.

FIGURE 4.10. ECONSULT.

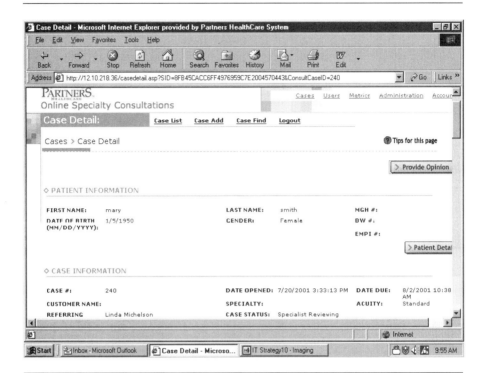

The fragile patient, such as a patient with congestive heart failure, will need all the same services, and in addition, there may need to be an application component that assists in monitoring the patient's medical status, such things as weight and blood oxygen saturation.

The plan that resulted can be summarized as follows:

• Conduct pilots of software to support the well patient. These pilots should determine patient satisfaction with the service and impact of the service on practice operations. Once pilots have been completed, the applications should be offered for broad implementation. Figure 4.11 provides an example of a patient requesting a medication refill through an application called PatientGateway.

• Pilots should be conducted for the chronically ill populations who have diabetes, epilepsy, and asthma. These pilots should assess the impact on patient health status and satisfaction with the care process. The pilots should seek to determine if a core application can be offered broadly across different populations with chronic disease or whether each population has very idiosyncratic needs. Payers should be invited to participate in the pilots to determine interest in covering this service.

FIGURE 4.11. PATIENT GATEWAY PRESCRIPTION REFILL.

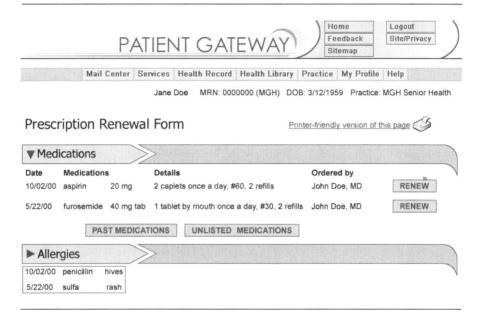

• Pilots should be conducted for congestive heart failure patients and chronic obstructive pulmonary disease patients. These pilots should seek to understand the contribution of the service to improved health status. Payers should be invited to participate in these trials as well.

Payer Relationships. There are three areas where the Internet may affect the interactions and relationships between providers and payers: insurance transactions, operational integration, and competing functions.

Providers and payers engage in a series of transactions that support their contractual relationship. These transactions include eligibility determination, referrals, and claims submission. The Internet can be used as a transaction "pipe," and Internet-based services such as transaction routing and translation can be offered. The ability to conduct these transactions electronically is a cornerstone of HIPAA and offers spectacular opportunities to reduce transaction costs and improve provider revenue capture.

However, even if all gains had been achieved through the use of electronic transactions, operational difficulties and inefficiencies can still plague the interactions between providers and payers. Providers may have imperfect knowledge of payer claims edits, leading to unnecessary claim rejections. Providers and payers may have different spellings or versions of a patient's name, for example, Beth and

Elizabeth, leading to needless claim rejections. Utilization review and medical management functions may be redundant. Payers and providers have an opportunity to reengineer the processes that bind them, perhaps involving the use of the Internet, and achieve further reductions in costs and gains in service quality.

The Web sites of both payers and providers may offer patient or subscriber services such as specialist consultation, health information, disease management protocols, personal health records, and prescription refill capabilities. The redundancy of these functions can lead to patient confusion and physician annoyance.

The plan that resulted from these observations can be summarized as follows:

• Implementation of Web-based support of electronic payer transactions should continue using the regional electronic data interchange infrastructure, the New England Healthcare EDI Network (NEHEN). Given the spectacular return on investment of this class of application, the implementation should be accelerated. Figure 4.12 depicts the NEHEN eligibility determination screen.

FIGURE 4.12. NEHEN ELIGIBILITY DETERMINATION.

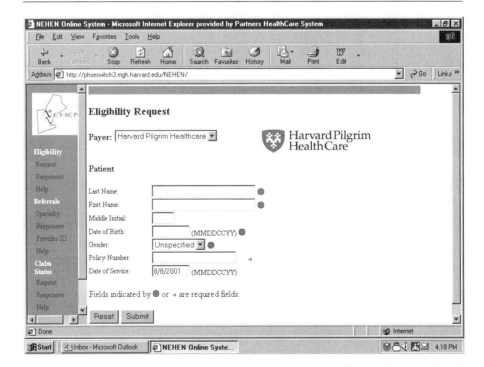

- Partners should engage in discussions with its major payers to identify areas where mutual operations can be streamlined and made more cost-effective. Initial conversations should focus on synchronizing member eligibility data, propagating claims edit logic throughout the Partners organization, and electronic remittance.

- Partners should initiate conversations with payers to develop guidelines and approaches to minimize the redundancy and confusion that may result from competing services being offered on respective Web sites. This may involve linking to Partners Web sites a "lite" version of payer Web sites from which conflicting information has been removed.

Marketing and Patient Channeling. The Internet is often seen as a mechanism to establish and extend brand identity. Customers generally develop a sense of an organization's brand through images a company projects, directly or indirectly, via mechanisms such as advertisements or articles about the company in the local newspaper. In addition, brand identity is based on customers' experiences with the company—for example, was the company responsive and courteous? Several health care dot-com companies developed portals involving cobranding, in which the brand of the dot-com, because of its image, might enhance the brand of the hospital. Provider organizations might see their Web site as a means to establish an image by providing information about services and enhance the customer experience by, for example, enabling requests for appointments or permitting the customer to "ask a specialist."

The Internet might also be used as a channeling mechanism, providing patients seeking care or health care services with another way of finding the organization. Channeling can happen because of image enhancement. It can also happen because a patient searching for treatments for a rare form of cancer finds that the organization offers such services. Channeling can happen because a conversation in a chat room recommends the organization to a patient newly diagnosed with a disease. Channeling can happen because of cross–Web site linkages, for example, a link to pediatric services from a site set up to help people who have recently moved to a new locality.

The value of the Internet as a mechanism to enhance brand or channel patients is unclear. It can be difficult to distill the impact of the Web site from other factors that affect brand, such as radio ads. It can be difficult to determine the extent to which new patients come to the organization because of the Internet. Web site hits can have little relationship to new business volume. Patients may cite the Web as part of their decision to seek care at an organization, but it can be unclear whether the Web site clinched the decision or merely supported the decision.

   The Partners plan in marketing and patient channeling had several recommendations:

• Overhaul existing hospital Web sites in an effort to improve the image they project and introduce basic service elements, such as the ability to request an appointment.

• Develop better metrics to track Web traffic and identify new patients whose health care decisions were influenced by the sites.

• Develop cross-linkages between sites throughout Partners—for example, a link from the stroke Web site at Massachusetts General Hospital to the stroke rehabilitation services of Spaulding Rehabilitation Hospital.

• Experiment with linkages to public or commercial Web sites to determine the degree of patient channeling that can result. Figure 4.13 provides an example of a link from America Online's Digital City to Brigham and Women's Hospital's site.

FIGURE 4.13. DIGITAL CITY–BRIGHAM AND WOMEN'S HOSPITAL LINK.

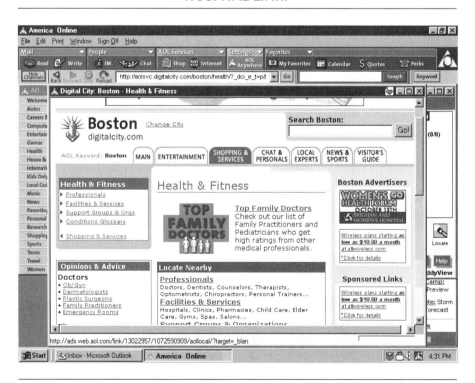

Summary: The Internet

Periodically, organizations must confront new technology with which they, and the industry, have little experience. Moreover, the organization may suspect that the technology has great potential and so recognizes that a lack of understanding is a problem.

When this occurs, the formation of view becomes very important. Two classes of view are needed, and both were illustrated in the discussion of the Internet.

For the first class, the organization develops an understanding of the possible meaning and contribution of the technology. Core capabilities, roles, categories of possible uses, and the futures that might be created enable the organization to develop a sense of what the technology might mean to their strategies, processes, and competitive position. The early experiences of others can be used to test and refine the organization's sense of meaning and contribution.

For the second class, the organization needs to develop a management philosophy and a set of guidelines that will shape its approach to the implementation of the technology if that is warranted. This philosophy can emphasize degrees of experimentation, the relative sense of urgency of adoption, the multifaceted (or nonmultifaceted) nature of the adoption, and the degree to which adoption will be subjected to analytical rigor, such as ROI analysis, or be couched as a strategic imperative.

In the discussion of the Internet, we saw strategy formulation (the definition of the nine categories of Internet leverage) and strategy implementation (the examples of an Internet plan for four categories). The sample plans hint at a range of changes to the IT asset: a Web-enabled infrastructure, the establishment of a function to manage remote consultations, and the adaptation of applications to support patient-provider communication.

Finally, the Internet discussion illustrated the situation in which a technology is assessed for strategic fit. The Internet plan was not derived from the strategies of Partners. Nor was it a broad response to a series of strategies. Rather the plan resulted from an assessment of the degree to which the Internet could be used to support existing strategies or open up new strategies.

The second opinion strategy illustrates several aspects of the Internet strategy discussion:

- The decision to pursue second opinions arose from several strategy directions, only one of which was the fit of the technology with the Partners strategic goal of leveraging its specialists.
- Second opinions are an example of service provision, and they leverage the service aspects of reach (to the globe) and efficiency of richness (less expensive access to a consulting physician).

- Due to the uncertainty of the future value of Internet-based second opinions, the strategy recommended a management response of a set of pilot efforts.
- There are elements of formulation (arriving at the conclusion of second opinion) and implementation (creation of a Web site and organizational unit).
- IT asset changes were required, including the eConsult application, staff to manage incoming consultation requests, and the placement of oversight of the project with the Partners Specialty Care Development Committee.

Summary

In this chapter, we discussed three examples of IT strategy: clinical information systems, integration, and the Internet.

The examples illustrated different aspects of linkage of IT strategy to organizational strategy. Clinical information systems can be derived directly from organizational strategies to improve patient care. Integration is a broad IT asset response to a range of delivery system integration efforts. The Internet is examined through the lens of organizational strategy to determine if the technology presents opportunities.

All of the examples involved strategy formulation and implementation. In the adverse drug event example, clinical information systems development centered on the idea of intervening at the time of ordering (formulation). A provider order entry application, medical informatics staff, and committees to manage system logic were established (implementation). The integration strategy developed a list of desired characteristics and capabilities (formulation) and the definition of the transcendent core (implementation). The Internet strategy developed a list of nine categories of use (formulation) and plans for each category (implementation).

The examples focused on leveraging core organizational processes: orders, accessibility of patient data across a continuum, and insurance transactions. There were also examples of improving the capture of critical data: order rationale, continuum quality measures, and Web-centric patient channeling. And there were examples of service differentiation; patient-provider interaction, and marketing.

All of the examples required changes and enhancements to the IT asset, including the following:

- Applications: provider order entry, clinical data repository, and payer electronic data interchange
- Data: coded problem lists, quality measurement data, and information on new business that resulted from Internet channeling efforts

- Infrastructure: a highly reliable and potent platform, a regional network, and Web application servers
- IT staff: medical informatics talent, medical imaging staff, and a remote consultation support function
- IT governance: Care Improvement Steering Committee, System Integration Committee, and Internet Strategy Committee

The three examples introduced the notion of view, the concepts and ideas that frame how any organization thinks about a strategic IT challenge. For clinical information systems, key view elements included the following:

- Clinical management of care and care as a process
- IT-centric improvement of care as an iterative activity focusing on care processes
- The creation of information-rich processes

For integration, key view elements included these:

- Constellations
- Transcendent processes
- Minimally invasive delivery of chunks

For the Internet, key view elements included the following:

- Four core technical capabilities
- Leverage of information distribution, service provision, and process extension
- An evolutionary, rather than revolutionary, impact

These views have great power, for they guide subsequent, significant decisions about the role of these technologies and applications, the organization's approach to their implementation and management, and the manner in which an organization evaluates the success of the technology.

Although view formation is a complex and frankly mysterious process, asking a small number of questions and thoughtfully developing answers can assist in ensuring that the view is well conceived.

CHAPTER FIVE

CONCLUSION

Health care organizations are making, and will continue to make, significant investments in information technology. They will do so in an effort to further organizational goals of improving care quality, reducing costs, enhancing service, growing market share, and perhaps transforming themselves into integrated delivery systems.

These efforts and investments can be thwarted or hindered by a myriad of problems and issues. However, the two core IT risks are the failure to conceptualize or develop a sound IT strategy and the failure to implement that strategy well. Strategy conceptualization failures may be the more significant of the two. A brilliant implementation of an incorrect strategy is not particularly helpful.

Strategy development permeates several aspects of IT: the linkage between organizational strategies and IT plans and activities, the development and advancement of internal IT capabilities and characteristics, and the elaboration of concepts or views that frame an organization's understanding of a major IT initiative, challenge, or technology, such as the role of the Internet.

The linking of organizational strategies to IT strategies and plans is complex. Frameworks and methodologies exist that can assist the development of the link between the two. Some frameworks help derive the IT strategy directly from organizational strategies. Other frameworks put forward core views of organizations—for example, the world can be defined in terms of value chains or competitive forces—from which IT opportunities can be discovered.

Although these frameworks and methodologies can be very helpful, linkage may always be difficult and fraught with problems. Evolving or incomplete strategies and imperfect understanding of IT opportunities are factors that get in the way.

A mature linkage process generally has the IT strategy discussion as an integral, ongoing component of the overall organizational strategy development process.

Health care organizations can draw from the lessons learned by others in their efforts directed toward applying IT to enhance the competitiveness of the organization. These lessons on IT-based competitiveness highlight the leverage that IT can provide to improving or reengineering critical core organization processes, capturing and reporting of critical data, delivering new or differentiated products and services, and even supporting the transformation of the basic culture and characteristics of the organization.

An IT-based competitive advantage is very difficult to sustain, although the sustainability is enhanced if IT leverages some other significant organizational strength such as having a large market share. In all cases, IT cannot overcome inadequate assessments of the environment, poor organizational strategies, weak management, or limited abilities to execute. The aggressive application of IT to improve a competitive position can also carry baggage such as a "permanent" increase in operating costs without a comparable increase in margins.

The IT asset is composed of applications, architecture, data, IT staff, and IT governance. These assets have characteristics and different ways of contributing to organizational performance. Often neglected, IT asset strategies must be developed. These strategies should be directed to ensuring that the ability of the organization to implement its IT plans is strong, robust, and improving.

In addition to the asset, IT effectiveness is also governed by intangible but real factors such as the relationship between IT and the rest of the organization and the chemistry between the CIO and other members of organizational senior leadership. Organizations must establish and nurture these intangible factors. These factors, along with the IT asset, may be the greatest contributor to an organization's ability to significantly effect IT-based contributions and to sustain those contributions over time.

As IT asset plans and strategies are developed, organizations should be wary of surveys, fads, and evaluation techniques, which can mislead as well as inform.

Poor linkage between IT strategy and organizational strategy, as well as inadequate IT asset development, can hinder the ability of an organization to realize value from its IT investments. Other factors also contribute to value dilution; examples include failure to state goals, failure to manage the delivery of value, inappropriate analyses applied to the investment proposal, and poor project management.

The strategies at Partners HealthCare System regarding clinical information systems, integration, and the Internet, were discussed in Chapter Four. Significant differences between these three areas of concern were quite clear: Clinical information systems were derived from a review of the overall strategy of care improvement. Integration was a broad asset response to a range of care integration strategies. The Internet was an example of a technology looking for a strategic fit.

Despite the differences, in all three cases, we saw changes to the IT asset. Strategies were necessary to define changes in applications, staff, data, architecture, and governance. In each of these areas, the component of the asset that represented the most challenging change varied.

In these examples, we also saw an emphasis on using IT to leverage organizational processes and data.

Finally, in these examples, we discussed the importance of the formulation of a view or governing concept of the IT strategy. For clinical information systems, this view resulted in the definition of the core of the IT response being the support of information-rich processes. Integration was defined in terms of concepts such as constellations and the transcendent core. The Internet was defined in terms of its leverage of information distribution and service. The formulation of this view can be guided by the answers to a small number of questions. The questions are easy to state; thoughtful answers are difficult to develop.

I hope that this book has been informative and perhaps enlightening. It is clear from my experience that IT can help effect very significant improvements in care and enhance the ability of health care provider organizations to thrive.

Too often, however, health care IT leaders immerses themselves in conversations about which vendor is the best at delivering a certain type of application, whether a component of technology such as handheld devices has promise or whether phenomena such as outsourcing offer real benefits. These conversations are not inappropriate; these areas require discussion and thought. But the conversations are incomplete. The effective and strategic application of IT in health care is a vastly broader and deeper challenge than these conversations would imply. Too narrow a focus does not serve well the organization's effort to craft IT-based effectiveness.

With this book, I hope to have advanced that effectiveness.

REFERENCES

Bates, D. W. Internal analysis, Partners HealthCare System, 1998.

Bates, D. W., and others. "Potential Identifiability and Preventability of Adverse Events Using Information Systems." *Journal of the American Medical Informatics Association*, 1994, *1*, 404–411.

Bates, D. W., and others. "Effect of Computerized Physician Order Entry and a Team Intervention on Prevention of Serious Medication Errors." *Journal of the American Medical Association*, 1998, *280*, 1311–1316.

Bell, C. W. "A Health Imperative." *Modern Healthcare*, Mar. 29, 1999, pp. 15–18.

Bensaou, M., and Earl, M. "The Right Mind-Set for Managing Information Technology." *Harvard Business Review*, Sept.-Oct. 1998, pp. 119–128.

Bresnahan, J. "What Good Is Technology?" *CIO Enterprise*, July 15, 1998, pp. 25–30.

Cash, J. I., Jr., McFarlan, F. W., and McKenney, J. L. *Corporate Information Systems Management: The Issues Facing Senior Executives*. Burr Ridge, Ill.: Irwin, 1992.

Cecil, J., and Goldstein, M. "Sustaining Competitive Advantage from IT." *McKinsey Quarterly*, 1990, *4*, 74–89.

Christensen, C. M. *The Innovator's Dilemma*. Boston: Harvard Business School Press, 1997.

Christensen, C. M. "The Past and Future of Competitive Advantage." *MIT Sloan Management Review*, 2001, *42*(2), 105–109.

College of Healthcare Information Management Executives. *The Healthcare CIO: A Decade of Growth*. Ann Arbor, Mich: College of Healthcare Information Management Executives, 1998.

Davenport, T. H. *Process Innovation: Reengineering Work Through Information Technology*. Boston: Harvard Business School Press, 1993.

Davenport, T. H., and Prusak, L. *Working Knowledge*. Boston: Harvard Business School Press, 1998.

Dell, M. *Direct from Dell.* New York: Harper Press, 1999.

Downes, L., and Mui, C. *Unleashing the Killer App.* Boston: Harvard Business School Press, 1998.

Drazen, E., and Metzger, J. *Strategies for Integrated Health Care.* San Francisco: Jossey-Bass, 1998.

Drazen, E., and Staisor, D. "Information Support in an Integrated Delivery System." *Proceedings of the 1995 Annual HIMSS Conference.* Chicago: Healthcare Information and Management Systems Society, 1995.

Drucker, P. F. *Management Challenges for the 21st Century.* New York: HarperBusiness, 2000.

Earl, M. J. "Experiences in Strategic Information Systems Planning." *MIS Quarterly,* 1993, *17*(1), 1–24.

Earl, M. J., and Feeny, D. F. "Is Your CIO Adding Value?" *McKinsey Quarterly,* 1995, *2,* 144–161.

Evans, P., and Wurster, T. S. *Blown to Bits: How the New Economics of Information Transforms Strategy.* Boston: Harvard Business School Press, 2000.

Feeny, D. F. "Making Business Sense of the E-Opportunity." *MIT Sloan Management Review,* 2001, *42*(2), 41–51.

Flammini, S. Internal analysis, Partners HealthCare System, 2001.

Freedman, D. "The Myth of Strategic IS." *CIO Magazine,* July 1991, pp. 42–48.

Gandhi, T., and others. "Satisfaction with the Referral Process from the Primary Care and Specialist Perspectives." *Journal of General Internal Medicine,* 1998, *13*(suppl.), 47.

GartnerGroup. *Defining a Flexible IT Architecture.* GartnerGroup Management Strategies and Directions Research Note SPA-03-3708. Stamford, Conn.: GartnerGroup, 1998a.

GartnerGroup. "GartnerGroup Research Notes SPA-TECH-050, KA-04-5517, QA-03–4925, TU-TECH-051, SPA-TECH-052." *CHIME Connection,* Sept. 1998b, pp. 4–12.

Glaser, J. P. "Managing the Management of Information Systems." *Healthcare Executive,* Jan.-Feb. 1991, pp. 12–15.

Glaser, J. P. "The Siren Call of the Slogan." *Healthcare Informatics,* July 1996, pp. 26–28.

Glaser, J. P. "Beware 'Return on Investment.'" *Healthcare Informatics,* June 1997, pp. 134–138.

Glaser, J. P., and Williams-Ashman, A. "Keeping the Database Healthy." *Information Week,* June 25, 1990, p. 72.

Harvard Business School. *Competitive Strategy: Articles from the* Harvard Business Review *and Case Studies from the Harvard Business School.* Boston: Harvard Business School Press, 1998.

Henderson, J. C., and Venkatraman, N. "Strategic Alignment: Leveraging Information Technology for Transforming Organizations." *IBM Systems Journal,* 1993, *32*(1), 4–16.

Herzlinger, R. *Market-Driven Health Care.* Reading, Mass.: Addison-Wesley, 1997.

Hopper, M. D. "Rattling SABRE: New Ways to Compete on Information." *Harvard Business Review,* May-June 1990, pp. 118–125.

"Internet Pioneers: We Have Lift-Off." *Economist,* Feb.3, 2001, pp. 69–72.

Keen, P.G.W. *The Process Edge.* Boston: Harvard Business School Press, 1997.

Kilbridge, P., and Drazen, E. "Information Systems for IDNs: Best Practices and Key Success Factors." *Proceedings of the 1998 Annual HIMSS Conference.* Chicago: Healthcare Information and Management Systems Society, 1998.

Lacity, M., and Willcocks, L. "An Empirical Investigation of Information Technology Sourcing Practices: Lessons from Experience." *MIS Quarterly,* 1998, *22,* 363–408.

Lake, K., Mehta, A., Adolf, R., and Hammarskjold, A. "Cashing In on Your ATM Network." *McKinsey Quarterly,* 1998, *1,* 173–178.

Leape, L., and others. "Systems Analysis of Adverse Drug Events." *Journal of the American Medical Association,* 1995, *274,* 35–43.

Le Grow, G., and others. *ASPs: An Executive Report*. Oakland: California HealthCare Foundation, 2000.

Levitin, A. V., and Redman, T. C. "Data as a Resource: Properties, Implications, and Prescriptions." *MIT Sloan Management Review*, 1998, *40*(1), 89–101.

Lipton, M. "Opinion: Demystifying the Development of an Organizational Vision." *MIT Sloan Management Review*, 1996, *37*(4), 83–92.

Malone, T. W., and Rockart, J. F. "Computers, Networks, and the Corporation." *Scientific American*, Sept. 1991, pp. 128–136.

Marietti, C. "Bullet-Proof Warehouses." *Healthcare Informatics*, Sept. 1998, pp. 41–50.

Martin, J., Wilkins, A., and Stawski, S. "The Component Alignment Model: A New Approach to Health Care Information Technology Strategic Planning." *Topics in Health Information Management*, 1998, *19*(1), 1–10.

McFarlan, F. W. "Information Technology Changes the Way You Compete." *Harvard Business Review*, May-June 1984, pp. 98–103.

McKenney, J. L., Copeland, D. G., and Mason, R. *Waves of Change: Business Evolution Through Information Technology*. Boston: Harvard Business School Press, 1995.

Minard, B. *Health Care Computer Systems for the 1990s: Critical Executive Decisions*. Chicago: Health Administration Press, 1991.

National Research Council. *Networking Health: Prescriptions for the Internet*. Washington, D.C.: National Academies Press, 2000.

National Research Council. *Building a Workforce for the Information Economy* Washington, D.C.: National Academies Press, 2001.

Pew Internet and American Life Project. *The Online Health Revolution*. Washington, D.C.: Pew Internet and American Life Project, 2000.

Porter, M. E. *Competitive Strategy*. New York: Free Press, 1980.

Porter, M. E. "Strategy and the Internet." *Harvard Business Review*, Mar.-Apr. 2001, pp. 63–78.

Porter, M. E., and Millar, V. E. "How Information Gives You a Competitive Advantage." *Harvard Business Review*, July-Aug. 1985, pp. 149–160.

Quinn, J. B., and others. *Information Technology in the Service Society*. Washington, D.C.: National Academy Press, 1994.

Roberts, P. "Client-Server at Brigham and Women's Hospital: An Enterprise of PCs." In R. Khanna (ed.), *Integrating Personal Computers in a Distributed Client-Server Environment*. Upper Saddle River, N.J.: Prentice Hall, 1995.

Ross, J. W., Beath, C. M., and Goodhue, D. L. "Develop Long-Term Competitiveness Through IT Assets." *MIT Sloan Management Review*, 1996, *38*(1), 31–42.

Sambamurthy, V., and Zmud, R. W. *Information Technology and Innovation: Strategies for Success*. Morristown, N.J.: Financial Executives Research Foundation, 1996.

Short, J. E., and Venkatraman, N. "Beyond Business Process Redesign: Redefining Baxter's Business Network." *MIT Sloan Management Review*, 1992, *34*(1), 7–21.

Sittig, D. Internal analysis, Partners HealthCare System, 1998.

Standage, T. *The Victorian Internet: The Remarkable Story of the Telegraph and the Nineteenth Century's On-Line Pioneers*. New York: Berkley, 1999.

Stern, C., and Stalk, G. (eds.). *Perspectives on Strategy*. New York: Wiley, 1998.

Strassmann, P. *The Business Value of Computers*. New Canaan, Conn.: Information Economics Press, 1990.

Strassmann, P. *The Squandered Computer*. New Canaan, Conn.: Information Economics Press, 1997.

Tapscott, D. *Blueprint to the Digital Economy.* New York: McGraw-Hill, 1998.

Teich, J. M. "Components of the Optimal Ambulatory Care Computing Environment." *Proceedings of the Ninth World Congress on Medical Informatics.* Edmonton, Alberta, Canada: International Medical Informatics Association, 1998.

Teich, J. M., and others. "Enhancement of Clinician Workflow Using Computer Order Entry." *Journal of the American Medical Informatics Association,* 1995, *2*(suppl.), 459–463.

Teich, J. M., and others. "Toward Cost-Effective Quality Care: The Brigham Integrated Computing Systems." *Proceedings of the Nicholas E. Davies CPR Recognition Symposium.* Chicago: Computerized Patient Record Institute, 1996.

Teich, J. M., and others. "Effects of Computerized Physician Order Entry on Prescribing Practices." *Archives of Internal Medicine,* 2000, *160,* 2741–2747.

"The 2001 HBR List: Breakthrough Ideas for Today's Business Agenda." *Harvard Business Review,* July-Aug. 2001, pp. 123–128.

Weill, P., and Broadbent, M. *Leveraging the New Infrastructure: How Market Leaders Capitalize on Information Technology.* Boston: Harvard Business School Press, 1998.

INDEX